VISION LOSS

Strategies for Living with Hope and Independence

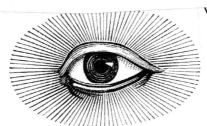

PEGGY R. WOLFE

Third Edition

PARK PUBLISHING, INC.
Minneapolis, Minnesota
New Richmond, Wisconsin

Third edition

Printed in the United States of America

ISBN: 978-0-9792945-3-2

Library of Congress Cataloging-in-Publication data
  Wolfe, Peggy R.
  [Macular disease]
  Vision loss : strategies for living with hope and independence / Peggy R. Wolfe. — 3rd edition.
       pages cm
  Previous editions published under the title: Macular disease.
  Includes index.
  ISBN 978-0-9792945-3-2
  1. Retinal degeneration--Popular works. 2. Low vision--Handbooks, manuals, etc. I. Title.
  RE661.D3W65 2014
  617.7'35—dc23

                                                        2013043428

Editor: Marly Cornell
Cover and interior designer: Monica Baziuk
Photography: Scott Knutson
Indexer: Galen Schroeder

Product photographs and trademarks are used in this book for informational purposes only. This book is not endorsed or sponsored by, or otherwise affiliated with, any of the manufacturers or trademark owners.

PARK PUBLISHING, INC.
511 Wisconsin Drive
New Richmond, Wisconsin 54017

Contents

Hope and Independence Intertwined

VISION LOSS: Strategies for Living with Hope and Independence is the 3rd edition of the book formerly named *Macular Disease: Practical Strategies for Living with Vision Loss*. The new title reflects my expanded understanding of the world of vision loss. I've learned from the people I've met that, no matter the cause or extent of our vision loss, we want to live with hope and maintain maximum independence.

"WE CAN DO IT" is the message of this book. Vision loss need not deter us. Maintaining a hopeful outlook nurtures our natural resilience and inspires us to find ways to live with as much independence as we can safely handle. Hope and independence are intertwined partners—each reinforces the other. The key to preserving our independence, even in the face of the challenges presented by declining vision, is to cultivate our resilience and the ability to sustain a hopeful spirit.

This book is written for all affected by vision loss, including families and friends who can gain insight and an understanding of the challenges faced by their loved ones, and doctors and other clinicians who can learn how their patients must cope from day to day.

My expertise comes from having lived with vision loss from macular degeneration since 1999. I do not attempt to address medical aspects of vision loss; rather, the book is a personal guide to dealing with actual situations and challenges.

I'm again writing in real time as I continue to adjust to the progressive decline of my own vision. When diagnosed with macular degeneration at the relatively "young" age of sixty-nine, I wasn't too surprised, as my mother and my uncle lived with macular disease for many years. They provided me with gutsy examples of how to live with vision loss.

Longtime exposure to their stalwart optimism left me with an accepting spirit—one filled not with fear, but with the will to do battle. At eighty-three, I'm still fighting my vision loss by finding strategies to make my life easier and by preparing for the day when I may have to rely solely on my peripheral vision.

Your life, after receiving a diagnosis of a vision disease, will likely take a different course than you expected. However, the information offered in this book demonstrates that the picture is not a hopeless one. You can still do the things you have been doing—though you may need to do them in different ways.

Those of us living with vision loss experience both trials and triumphs, and some of mine are illustrated here in the form of personal stories. Each chapter in this book also offers practical strategies for everyday life. You can use ideas in this book that have worked for others to find solutions that work for you.

Parents of a child with vision loss can gain insight and learn about vision rehabilitation and a variety of resources. I direct you especially to the National Association for Parents of Children with Visual Impairments (NAPVI). See description in Appendix B.

My goal in writing this book is to share what I have learned from my experience and from others in the same situation. By finding tactics to deal with the realities of declining vision and embarking on a strategic game plan—we need not be "victims" of our vision loss. We can be victors and have an independent and fulfilling life. There is hope, and there is help.

Nourish the Spirit

WHAT DO WE MEAN BY "SPIRIT"? People think of spirit in many different ways. One definition is "life force." Helpful qualities within that concept include backbone, boldness, character, dauntlessness, energy, enterprise, enthusiasm, grit, guts, heart, humor, morale, motivation, resolve, soul, vitality, warmth, and will. Developing these inner resources will help you sustain a rewarding and independent life full of hope, courage, resilience, and purpose.

Develop positive attitudes and resilience

Consider the following qualities as gifts to help you develop the strong spirit that leads to a positive hopeful outlook: acceptance and patience, powerfulness, enthusiasm and enjoyment, and most important—gratitude. Think of how you can use these qualities to enhance your day-to-day life and develop resilience. I think of resilience as the ability to adjust to the changes and challenges we meet with vision loss by using our inner strength and outer resources.

Acceptance and patience

Realize that life involves change, and living with vision loss will include limitations you didn't expect. You may need to allow yourself to grieve your losses as you move toward acceptance. Understand that you are dealing not only with the loss of vision, but also the loss of what you thought the rest of your life might be like. As with any other grief, you may feel shock or disbelief, or even find yourself in denial that this is happening to you. Anger, fear, and questions of "Why me?" are common reactions. Certain everyday things may take longer to accomplish. You will be able to meet such new challenges more effectively if you can nurture a sense of calm and patience.

─────────────── **MY STORY** ───────────────

Spillovers and Knockovers

As my vision declined, I found it more and more difficult to see the level of coffee in the cup as I was

2

pouring. I had frequent spillovers, which made me frustrated, impatient, and mad at myself. I also knocked over my glass more often, spilling milk all over the table—and sometimes my chair and the floor.

I finally decided to allow myself one spillover or knockover per day. Now I've accepted that I will have these incidents. When I have a day with no such accident, I feel elated at having such a "good" day. When I do spill or knock something over, it's fine with me, because that's my expected allotment for the day. So I don't feel angry or impatient with myself anymore. On the rare occasion that I have two accidents—I just assign one to the next day!

———————————

Powerfulness

Many things in life are, and always have been, beyond our control—from the forces of nature to the behavior of others. Being confronted with some new limitations does not mean you are suddenly less powerful. Know that you still have control over how you live your life. There are still many parts of life that you can control. The most important thing you have a choice about is your attitude. When you are discouraged, counter that feeling with a determination to rule your own life. Since diseases affecting vision often have a slow progression, you may well have years of quite functional, albeit declining, vision. Consider such a diagnosis an "advance notice"—a gift of time to gradually prepare for the day that could come when you might have to rely only on limited peripheral or central vision. This book serves as a guide to things you can do in various areas of your life to bolster your confidence, sense of power, and ability to maintain your independence.

Enthusiasm and enjoyment

Be good to yourself, and do what is most important to you. At first, most people who receive a diagnosis of a vision disease feel confused, frightened, and depressed. I suggest that the first thing to do in that uncertain time is to figure out what things in your life bring you the most contentment and joy. Then immediately make plans to do one of these things as a special treat to yourself. Choose something that fills your heart with great joy. Practical activities required for daily living don't qualify. What you pick need not involve a financial expenditure, but rather the investment and the reward of love and time well spent. Take a walk with a friend in a beautiful park, or visit someone you haven't seen in a long time. Enjoy a museum, or go to a concert, or play with a friend.

You can save most of your ideas for later times, but this first one should be something really special. Then make a decision to find ways to be good to yourself on a continuing basis. Find ways to relax and have fun. If you want to meet people and learn new things, check out activities offered in your local area, such as community and senior centers—sign up for their newsletters and monthly calendars. Local low vision agencies offer classes and group excursions.

Maybe your idea of fun and relaxation is simply a slower pace to your life, so you can savor each day. Keep in touch with friends and relatives, play games on the Internet. Most important, be good to yourself.

Gratitude

Perhaps the most important quality of all is gratitude. Think of things in your life for which you are thankful.

I am thankful for—

- living for seventy years before the diagnosis of early macular disease.

- the gift of time to find ways to remain as independent as possible.

- willingness to ask for help when needed (still hard for me).

- family and friends who graciously help with tasks and transportation.

- injections in my right "good" eye that stopped bleeding.

- continued research into the treatments and cures for eye diseases.

- the inspiring people I've met in my local chapter of the Foundation Fighting Blindness.

Coping with grief and stress from loss of vision

Emotional reactions upon diagnosis may include a profound sadness. Many people have trouble dealing with anxiety about the future. These are normal and understandable emotions, and allowing yourself to feel them can help you to accept what is happening and then let go of your fears. If vision loss—which perhaps comes on top of other losses—causes you significant depression, it may help you, as it has helped many others, to seek counseling or join a vision loss support group. Be patient and gentle with yourself as you strive for acceptance every new day— it will bring both peace and the will to move forward to your "new normal" life.

Stress is a common reaction to vision loss. Taking twice as long to perform a simple task or beginning to acknowledge that you should stop driving are typical stressors. The body frequently expresses stress in the form of headaches, stomachaches, or trouble sleeping. When you feel particularly harried or frustrated or sad, try these stress-reducing methods:

- Take a break.
- Talk about it. If you are alone, call a family member or friend. The important thing is to talk about it.
- Tell someone if you are overwhelmed or need help, rather than wonder why others can't or don't see that you need help.

- Recognize that a grief expressed is a grief diminished.

- Know that it's okay to yell or cry.

- Realize that stress is contagious—if you feel stressed, chances are good that those around you will begin to feel stressed. Trying to ignore, deny, or bottle up feelings can result in a group of inwardly seething, frustrated people.

- Help someone else.

The best way to prevent stress from building up is, of course, to prevent it from taking hold in the first place. Here are some ways to ward off stress.

- Know your limits. Set realistic goals when planning your day.

- Be patient and accepting of yourself.

- Take frequent breaks by stretching and deep breathing.

- Refuse to hold grudges or feel sorry for yourself.

- Get enough sleep.

- Exercise regularly.

- Meditate or engage regularly in spiritual practices consistent with your beliefs.

- Laugh often, even if you don't feel like doing so. Smiling relaxes the muscles in your face.

———————————— **MY STORY** ————————————

Dream Trip after a Scary Prognosis

When my retinologist told me his guess that I had one to two years before I'd lose my central vision, I sat down and thought about how this new situation would affect my life—what I might be losing that mattered most. I decided the first step was to figure out what was most important to me. My answer was twofold—first, to spend time with my daughter, who lives in another state; and second, to experience the great joys of my life—classical music, opera, ballet, and visual arts. So I immediately planned a trip with my daughter to New York City. We shared all expenses, which helped to make our trip possible. We visited art museums and attended opera and ballet performances. I will always have the memory of our special time together doing things we both love.

————————————

Nurture your mind

Keep your mind active by reading. Chapter 4 is devoted to the many ways to read, from large print books to electronic books to "listening" to books. Listening is a skill that becomes increasingly handy as vision declines. Listening to the radio or TV with your eyes closed helps to develop those skills.

Learn something new. Adult enrichment classes offered by your school district can exercise your mind as well as your body. Consider classes offered by community education organizations and low vision agencies. If you are not already using a computer, start now. Developing computer skills will open untold doors for you, and technological advances in accessibility are making computers easier and easier to use.

Find a spiritual home

For many people, belonging to a faith community brings spiritual fulfillment and peace. Membership in churches, synagogues, mosques, or other places of worship can lead to fellowship with others who can provide comfort and support. Many faith communities offer study groups and classes. If you do not already have such a spiritual home, but feel a yearning, seek out this type of supportive community.

Meet others with vision loss

Getting to know others with vision loss is reassuring and inspiring. You are not alone, and your hope will be replenished by learning how others navigate their lives. I am fortunate that there is a local chapter of the Foundation Fighting Blindness in my hometown. Knowing our members has transformed my life. I've met inspiring people of all ages with eye diseases I didn't even know existed. Learning that we all share the same challenges led me to write this new edition aimed at all those with vision loss.

Ask your doctor what vision organizations and agencies are available in your community. Some offer support groups and a variety of other services.

Volunteer for rich rewards

Perhaps the best thing to do for yourself, while helping others at the same time, is to become a volunteer. Churches, the United Way, senior centers, and other nonprofit organizations need volunteers for all types of jobs. Think about your skills and what you enjoy doing, and make a call. If there is a vision loss organization in your community, you can join an advocacy group or work with a staff member in a support group. The possibilities are endless.

——— MY STORY ———

A New Church, a Perfect Volunteer Job

I had been halfheartedly looking for a spiritual home for many years. I'd attend one church for a few months, then another. I did not feel at home in any of them. Then one Sunday, I attended a service at a church I'd been hearing had beautiful music. I had not gone there before, because I thought it was too huge a congregation. But as soon as I felt the friendly atmosphere and heard the soloist and choir, I knew this was where I belonged. My search was over. I joined the church right away. Soon I wanted to be more closely involved in its community, so I started looking for a volunteer job among the many offerings.

One day the coordinator called, said there was an opening in the music library, and asked if I'd be interested, considering I had a library degree. I said yes, and was soon working with a special woman who has become my "volunteer buddy." Our ongoing project was to list in a database each track of the hundreds of compact discs held by members of the music department. Our trio (coordinator and two volunteer buddies) has developed a close and loving relationship that is important to each of us. My friendship with these two women has enriched my life beyond words. The bonus is that I'm working with music, too. These have been great gifts to me.

———————

Eye Care

MONITOR YOUR VISION regularly. You are the one who is best able to identify small changes in your vision. Develop a proactive approach, and take fast action if you notice any sudden change. That may require immediate treatment. This is an important way to take care of your eyes and to keep seeing at the highest possible level.

Home vision tests

Annual checkups are not enough if you have macular degeneration. You must be responsible for monitoring your sight on a regular basis. You can do simple tests at home. Your eye doctor may have directed you to use an Amsler grid to check your own eyes periodically. Make the grid test a habit by doing it in the same location, with the same lighting, and at about the same time of day, so you can more accurately compare your results with those of previous tests. Be aware of what you see with each eye in order to notice any changes since the previous test.

There are other important ways to monitor your sight. Develop your own benchmark system. For example, you can test your vision by looking, with each eye, at a bedside clock, your watch, or the bathroom scale, or by reading with each eye to see if the lines are wavy or if your field of vision has narrowed. Choose something that you read every day or at least every week, such as a TV guide, a newspaper, or church program. Take note if you suddenly need more light for a particular task or if you develop a new sensitivity to glare. If you notice a change, see your eye doctor right away.

There is successful treatment for the wet form of macular degeneration and, at the time of this writing in 2013, promising research is underway for treatment of the dry form. Stem cell and gene therapies are promising new treatments for a variety of degenerative retinal diseases, such as retinitis pigmentosa, Stargardt disease, and Usher syndrome.

See the final chapter, Research Changes the Future, for more information.

Contact your doctor if you notice a change in either eye

- Act immediately, in time for helpful treatment.

- If you have trouble getting an immediate appointment, be an advocate for yourself and keep insisting that you see the doctor.

- Do not procrastinate!

Seeing things that aren't there? Charles Bonnet syndrome (CBS)

Don't be scared if you suddenly start seeing things that you know are not really there. This condition was identified and named by Swiss philosopher Charles Bonnet in 1760. His grandfather was almost blind, yet would state that he saw people, figures, buildings, and birds that he knew were not there.

The images are called visual hallucinations, and there are no accompanying voices or sounds, smells, or tastes. CBS is not a mental illness. The hallucinations are easily distinguishable from what is real even though they fit into the environment, such as children riding their bicycles down your street.

The images are the result of the brain's reaction to severe vision loss, usually from age-related diseases such as macular degeneration, diabetic retinopathy, cataracts, and glaucoma. When the symptoms first occur, the images often come frequently, maybe several times a day, but eventually diminish.

Characteristics of Bonnet syndrome include—

- hallucinations consisting of familiar images of people, animals, buildings, plants, trees, patterns (such as mosaics or lines) lasting for a few seconds, few minutes, or a couple of hours, over a period of weeks to years.

- possible initial misdiagnosis of early dementia or psychosis.

- spontaneous remission.

The frequency of hallucinations is sometimes reduced by staying physically and mentally occupied, spending time with family or friends, and participating in social activities.

Bring up the subject of Charles Bonnet syndrome to your family now, so they know about the symptoms before they could appear, and understand that these hallucinations are not a cause for worry. If there is concern, make an appointment to see your eye doctor to learn more about the disease. The best treatment is knowledge and reassurance. A positive attitude is the key.

Visit your eye doctors regularly for checkups and tests

When dealing with eye disease, it is important to have complete eye examinations every year. For retinal diseases, visit a specialist in retinal in diseases, a retinologist. You may be directed to have more frequent appointments. See an ophthalmologist on an annual basis for a general eye checkup and for a possible adjustment to the prescription for your eyeglasses.

When you go out of town, carry a copy of your eyeglass prescriptions, along with the phone numbers of your ophthalmologist, your retinologist, and the store where you purchased the glasses, in case you lose or break your glasses. If you have a sudden change in vision when you are away, be prepared to call your eye doctor for advice and a possible referral to a doctor in the vicinity. For a longer stay away from home, be prepared with the name and contact information of a eye doctor your doctor recommends. The new doctor can call your regular eye doctor to obtain your history, including treatments you have received.

At eye appointments, your distance vision is checked by reading rows of letters on a distant chart. Near vision may be checked by reading from a small card you hold in your hand that has rows of text or numbers in decreasing sizes of type. This card tests the vision for reading and other close work. If you have macular degeneration, you may be asked to check your eyes with an Amsler grid, like you use at home. These vision tests are usually followed by a glaucoma test. You are given drops to dilate your pupils so the doctor can see into the back of your eyes.

Depending on your diagnosis, further tests may be conducted. At an initial visit, two types of photographs may be taken with a special camera. One type takes color photos. The other is fluorescein angiography, which involves injecting a dye into a vein in your hand or arm. As the dye circulates through the bloodstream and eventually reaches the eye, the blood vessels in the retina become visible to the special camera, which takes flash photographs of the eye every few seconds for several minutes. These photo sessions can be uncomfortable due to the bright light that is flashed into your eyes, but the photos help the doctor determine changes or identify abnormal blood vessels. The fine detail shown in the photos, when enlarged, makes the fluorescein angiography an accurate and valuable tool for the diagnosis of many eye conditions.

Another test, called ocular coherence tomography (OCT), but informally called a scan, obtains high-resolution cross-sectional images of the retina. This is used to diagnose a host of macular diseases and to follow up on responses to various types of treatment. For example, if you have macular degeneration and bleeding is suspected, or if you have had injections in your eye, you will probably have OCT scans at each visit. The scans take just moments, and there is no discomfort as there are no bright flashes of light.

Shortly after the tests, the doctor visually examines your eyes, and checks and explains your test results.

Having someone present with you is an advantage so that you do not miss something important. Come prepared with a written list of questions, and take notes of the doctor's responses to your questions for later review. It is easy to forget details when there is a lot of information. Ask your companion to write down information the doctor gives about results of your tests, possible treatments, and suggestions for home care. At my own visits, a number of different people have come as my support person—my husband, son, daughter, and a cousin from Ireland who also had an appointment. These visits also help your family members understand your disease and how it is progressing.

MY STORY

Bleeding in the Right Eye— Then the Left?

I used to think the telltale sign of bleeding in the eye would be some wild vision distortion, such as seeing a twisted clock face or blurred crooked lines in a book or newspaper. But my retinologist always ended each visit by asking that I call if I noticed even a small change in either eye.

On my seventy-seventh birthday, I was feeling confident because I'd passed the vision test for renewing my driver's license two weeks earlier, much to my surprise. Yet I was trying not to admit to myself that something had changed in my right ("good") eye. That Sunday at church, where I gratefully use the large print program, I found for the first time that I could not read the ends of lines or see the music to sing. At home, glare from my computer screen had become intense. I had to change to different types of light bulbs in the dining room, where I have my morning coffee while I read the newspaper—which had suddenly become quite blurry with wavy lines. I was in the habit of testing my vision by reading the daily paper first with one eye, then the other. I usually did vision checks throughout each day, too, by looking at stationary distant objects. So I was able to pinpoint the problem to my right eye.

I was afraid to make the call to the doctor, but my son's words about the importance of caring for my vision kept ringing in my ears. I made the call after a few days.

My retinologist looked at my dilated right eye and said he saw bleeding, the sign that I now had wet macular degeneration. He ordered a fluorescein angiogram and an OTC scan, which confirmed the diagnosis. The doctor said he was surprised, and that I was young to have developed the wet form of macular degeneration. He said he was amazed that I'd noticed the change because the bleeding was so slight. He bemoaned the people who don't notice changes or put off seeing a doctor for six months—at which point, treatment is less able to help.

Before I left the office, treatment was started. I received an injection of Avastin in my right eye that we hoped would halt the bleeding so that my sight would stay at its present level. Almost immediately, my vision actually improved. When I went for my six-week checkup and another injection, we found that my vision had improved to the point that it had been before the bleeding. At the twelve-week point, my vision had continued to improve. I had another injection, as planned. At the six-month point, my right eye vision remained stable. I had no further bleeding until three years later, in 2010, when I then had a series of fifteen monthly Avastin injections. Each month, the OTC scan showed improvement and, finally, I was able to discontinue the injections.

My left eye has not developed bleeding, but degeneration of the cells in the macula has continued to accelerate. The eye is at a point far past the definition of "legal" blindness.

Special vitamins for macular degeneration

The National Eye Institute's "Age-Related Eye Disease Study" resulted in a vitamin supplement known as the AREDS formula. There are different varieties of the AREDS formula. The original formula contained beta-carotene (vitamin A), but not lutein (another naturally occurring carotenoid that aids in eyesight). A newer formula called AREDS2 contains lutein, but not beta-carotene. The National Eye Institute released the results of the five-year study of AREDS 2 in May 2013. This follow-up to the Age-Related Eye Disease Study (AREDS), studied the effect of adding lutein, zeaxanthin, and omega-3 to the original formula. The results show that lutein and zeaxanthin may be helpful, but omega-3 did not have a positive effect over five years. Ask your doctor which formula is right for you.

Sisters in Separate Studies

When I was diagnosed at my first visit in 1999, the retinologist told me about a research study that was testing low-level laser surgery as a way to slow the progress of macular degeneration. When he asked if I'd like to join the study, I immediately agreed. I've always been interested in research; and I knew that, even if it didn't help me, it could help others. I was the third patient in the practice to sign on. After I qualified for the study, the doctor received a sealed envelope that held a piece of paper with my name and either "Right eye" or "Left eye." I was hoping it would be my left eye that had been randomly selected because the right eye had better vision. But the patient had no choice, and my right eye was chosen. Following the laser treatment, my eyes were checked every six months for five years by a research coordinator who did special tests.

The results of multiple studies of low-level laser treatment showed no statistical advantage over not receiving any treatment.

As it happened, my sister was a participant at the same time in the AREDS study that tested the particular vitamin-antioxidant combination in the AREDS formula. It was this study that showed positive results. Taking the special formula slowed the progress of macular disease in some cases. Doctors then started to recommend taking AREDS pills on a daily basis.

Protect your eyes from the sun

It is generally a good idea to protect your eyes from the sun. If you are affected by glare, such protection is necessary for your comfort. Glare is also a problem for some people when they are in a car and even when indoors. Wide-brimmed and visor hats and sunglasses can provide protection.

Your doctor may recommend a certain type of sunglasses, or you may order from a low vision catalog. NoIR sunglasses are an inexpensive brand that comes in both fit-over and wraparound styles. They offer 100 percent ultraviolet protection. They also help prevent glare and block blue light. The wraparound model, shown on the next page, is excellent because it blocks sunlight from the sides. The sunglasses are reasonably priced and come in various sizes and lens colors. The color to select depends on your eye condition, as different colors are recommended for diabetic retinopathy, macular degeneration, and retinitis pigmentosa. Visit the NoIR website to see photos of the various colors available. A large selection of NoIR sunglasses is available through the low vision stores listed in Appendix A, and some of these stores have catalogs with helpful charts showing suitable sunglasses colors for various eye diseases. These low vision stores carry many other useful products, and you'll find many references to them throughout the book. I suggest you order a catalog right now.

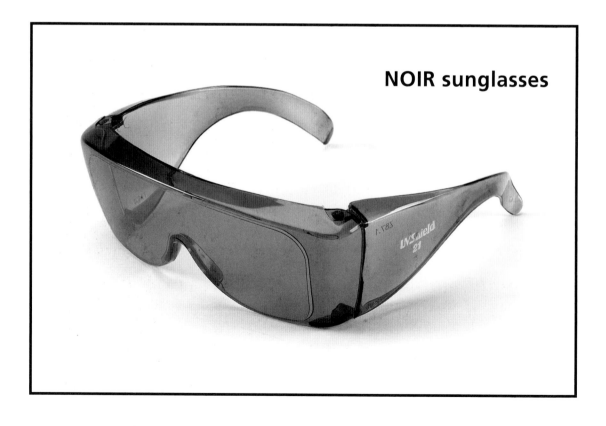

NOIR sunglasses

Get both reading and distance glasses

Having the proper glasses for both near-sight activities (such as reading, writing checks, and sewing) and far-sight activities (such as driving and watching television) allows you to have maximum field of vision at both far and close distances. If you currently wear bifocal or trifocal glasses, you may benefit from separate reading and distance glasses. I also have "computer" glasses that are set for the distance between my eyes and the computer monitor.

Keep your glasses clean

A smudge on your glasses can cause a big scare. Often when I start to read, it seems that my vision has suddenly gone. But when I hold my glasses up to the light, I see smudges and specks. I wear my reading glasses on a chain around my neck, and the way the lenses hang down seems to make them a magnet for specks and dust. I clean the lenses frequently and place bottles of glasses cleaner in every room, so it is easy to clean my glasses. Get tall bottles so you'll be able to spot them standing upright.

Fix drooping eyebrows and eyelids with surgery

As we age, upper eyelids sometimes droop and block the upper field of vision. This can give the appearance of half-open eyes. One cause of drooping is reduced tone in the muscles that control the eyelids. This condition can also be caused by eyebrows that droop so much that they make the eyelids droop as well. If this eyebrow drooping limits your field of vision, Medicare may cover approved surgical procedures to correct the problem. A direct brow lift fixes drooping eyebrows and is a fairly simple procedure. It is not the same as a forehead lift—a procedure that is done for cosmetic purposes is expensive and is not covered by Medicare.

If your eyelids themselves are drooping, understand that the surgery required to correct that problem is much more complicated. Talk to your eye doctor and consider your options carefully before proceeding.

—————————— MY STORY ——————————

Seeing Better and Looking Younger

In 2001 my visual field became severely obstructed by drooping eyelids, and my doctor sent me to an ophthalmic plastic surgeon for evaluation. His diagnosis was that my eyebrows were drooping so much that they made my eyelids droop. He took digital photos and sent them to my health insurer to see if my condition met the guidelines at that time for Medicare coverage in my state. The answer was yes, and I had a simple procedure called a "direct brow lift," in which excess skin from my forehead was removed in a wrinkle above my eyebrows. I felt fine and went to a cookout the next day, wearing sunglasses that covered my eyebrows. No one was the wiser.

A few weeks after surgery, the "after" photos were compared with the photo taken before surgery. The difference was startling, and the wrinkles above my eyebrows looked no more prominent than before the surgery. There were tiny scars; but, as they were right in the wrinkles, they were barely noticeable and faded away with time. I've retained my "younger," wide-eyed look all these years, and having a full field of vision has been helpful as my sight has declined.

––––––––––––––

3

Lighting for Essential Contrast

A WELCOME SURPRISE may be in store for you if reading is becoming an increasingly difficult and frustrating experience. Everyone needs more light to read as they grow older, but the need is especially great with low vision. Sometimes, being able to see better is simply a matter of properly placed, adequate lighting.

Indirect and direct lighting

There are two types of lighting. Ambient indirect lighting comes from ceiling fixtures and sunlight. It provides general light for an entire room. Direct task lighting provides the contrast needed for reading and close work by aiming light directly toward the task. This provides the contrast required to distinguish the letters in words and the type from the paper on which it is printed.

Ambient light is especially needed for safe passage around living spaces when it is dark outside. Ceiling fixtures provide the indirect light needed for general seeing. This lighting is turned on and off with a wall switch, preferably with a face plate that is a different color than the wall. Task lighting from portable lamps—floor, table, and task lamps—are good sources of direct lighting.

Choosing lamps to fit the task

Portable lamps come in many styles, from tall floor lamps to short task lamps, and with and without magnifiers. Floor lamps come with and without direct lighting. Torchiere floor lamps provide good general lighting that is easy on the eyes because it is indirect, with the light directed upward by a bulb in a reflecting bowl. Some models have a second, lower lamp on the pole that can give direct light for reading. Inexpensive models of such torchiere lamps are available in many chain stores.

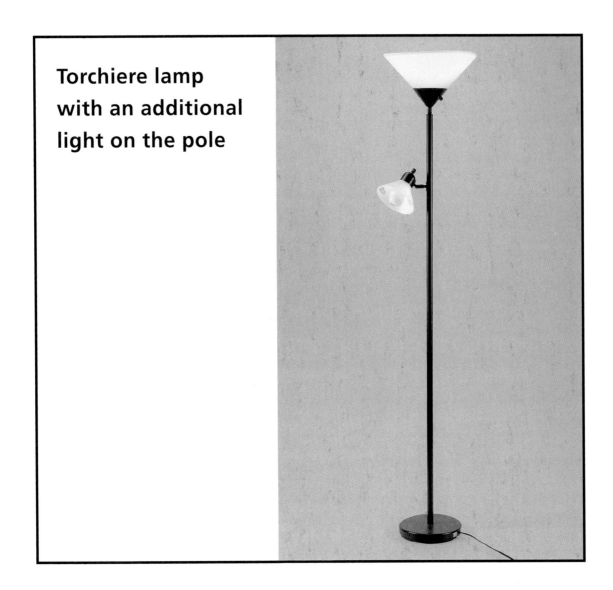

Torchiere lamp
with an additional
light on the pole

Floor and tabletop lamps with magnifiers

A more substantial and expensive type of lamp has a magnifying lens attached, either at the light source or on a separate arm. These lamps allow hands to remain free for reading and performing tasks. The lamps come in both table and floor models, which accommodate various types of light bulbs.

A Giraffe™ lamp with a rimless magnifier on the end of an adjustable arm is shown in the photo. This lamp

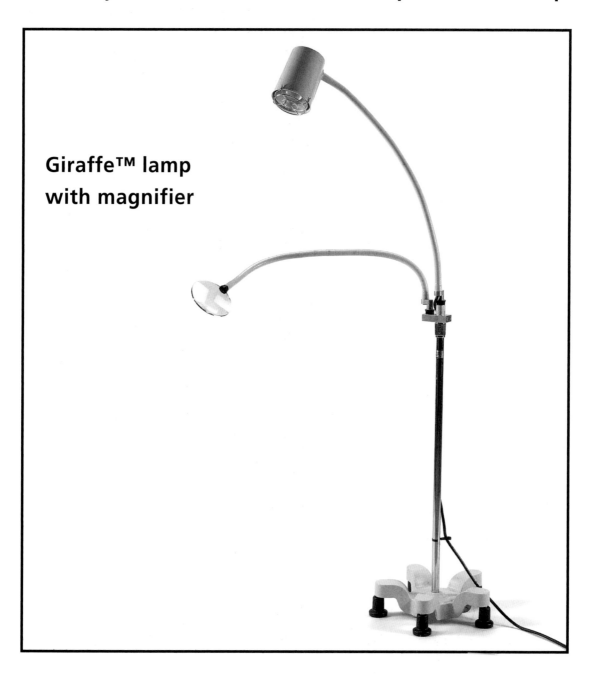

Giraffe™ lamp
with magnifier

has a 30" flexible gooseneck and a stationary anti-tip base. The height adjusts from 2 to 7 feet. This is a particularly useful floor lamp, because the long neck can easily be twisted to direct the light.

The first item I bought when my vision declined to the point that I needed better lighting (two-and-a-half years after my diagnosis) was a Giraffe lamp without the magnifier. I especially like this lamp because I can easily swing it around to where I want it, and bend it up or down as needed. As an extra bonus, the lamp swivels. Many other brands and models of lamps with magnifiers are available from low vision stores.

Desk and tabletop lamps

Traditional table lamps with lampshades do not provide a way to direct light where needed to read or perform tasks such as writing checks or other close work. When selecting a lamp for a table or desk, choose one with a flexible gooseneck that can be turned to direct light where needed. Reasonably priced small lamps, like the one shown in the photo on page 38, can be found in office supply and discount stores. Look for a lamp that comes with a halogen bulb for really strong light. Place task lamps to your

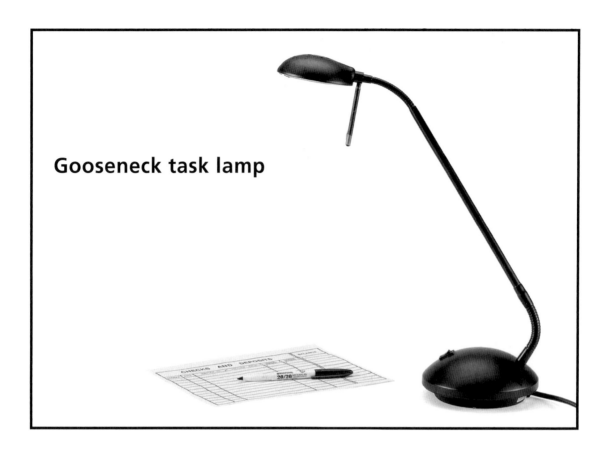

Gooseneck task lamp

side to avoid reflected glare from your work surface. Avoid looking directly at a bare bulb that is turned on. The handiest place I've put a small lamp is on my kitchen counter. I can see what I'm chopping and cooking, and I can turn the light to shine on my stove.

Magnifying task lamps

For even brighter task viewing, consider a magnifying lamp. This type of lamp has a high-intensity bulb and powerful magnification. These lamps cost less than the magnifying floor models.

Spot lighting with clip-on lamps

When you need to aim light at a particular spot, use a small lamp that directs the light right at the object you want to see. I use a clip-on lamp with a bendable neck above my microwave oven, positioned so that it shines light on the oven's buttons. When I first bought this oven, I could easily read the buttons' white numbers on the black background; but after a couple of years, I could no longer detect them—the entire control panel appeared black. The small light allows me to easily see the numbers once again. I use small 15" clip-on lights attached to my computer stand and aim the light at the keyboard so I can see the letters. Another is attached to the headboard of my bed. These inexpensive lamps are widely available in discount and home center stores. These lamps use halogen bulbs that give direct, bright light.

Flashlights

Perhaps the most indispensable type of light is the flashlight. LED flashlight models give bright light that is stronger than models using regular bulbs. LED flashlights are more expensive; but, for the brightest light, they are worth the extra cost. These small flashlights fit in a purse or pocket and have many uses.

Handy places to keep flashlights

- In the car—a must
- In the kitchen, to help find things in the refrigerator and in cupboards
- By your bed, to help you when you get up at night
- In your purse, briefcase, or pocket—indispensable at dimly lit restaurants, for reading the menu, and propped up for seeing your food
- By thermostats, if you need to adjust the settings
- By chairs and tables, so that you can find things that fall
- On your bureau, to help you see contents of drawers and locate items

Never leave home without a flashlight!

Lantern-style flashlights for power outages

Lantern-style flashlights provide strong lighting during power outages. Three models are shown here.

They each have a handle that makes them easy to carry; but even so, it is a good idea to have two or three lanterns that you can place in various rooms in the event of a power outage. Designate a specific place to keep the lanterns when they're not in use so they are easily accessible in the dark. I have three lanterns of different styles, and I keep them on top of the refrigerator. I know I can always find an object that large, even in the dark. I position each of my lanterns with the handle facing outward so I don't have to grapple in the dark to pick one up.

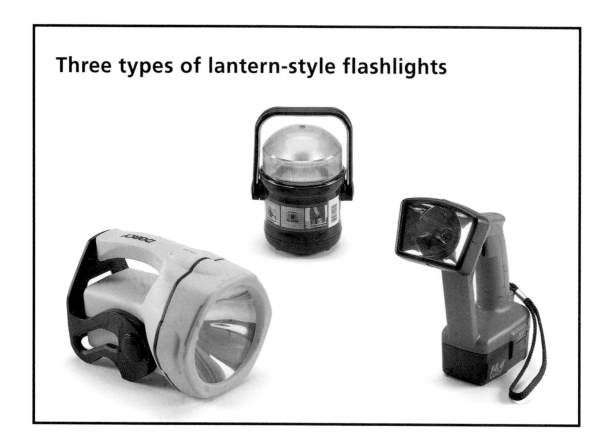

Three types of lantern-style flashlights

Nightlights

Although not for reading, nightlights are indispensable for helping you find your way in the dark. Put one in your bedroom, bathroom, hallways, and any other areas where you are likely to walk at night. Also, have a beacon by your bed, such as a lighted clock on a bedside table.

Choosing light bulbs by color ratings

Color temperature is a method of describing the characteristics of light, either warm (yellowish to orange to red) or cold (blue to violet). The most appropriate light bulbs for someone with vision loss will emit a warm color.

Color temperature determines a color rating. Ratings are located on the light bulb package. Look for "Lighting Facts," sometimes in a white block on the side or back of the package. "Light Appearance" will be near the end of the listings. Measurements are stated in degrees of Kelvin (°K), such as 2700 K. The lower the number, the warmer the color; the higher the number, the cooler the color.

Compact fluorescent, LED, and halogen bulbs are available in warm color ranges. Incandescent bulbs have warm ratings also, but will no longer be manufactured after the year 2014. The best bulbs to select will be in the warm color range of 2600 Kelvin to 3500 Kelvin. Because cold bluish light can be harmful to the eyes, look for bulbs in the warm color range.

How Contrast Is My Best Friend

Contrast provided by light enables me to see objects that seem to fade into the background. The greater the contrast, the easier it is to see things, from print on a page to peas on a plate. Adequate lighting is essential to provide the contrast required to distinguish items from their backgrounds. The use of contrast is so important when dealing with diminished vision that hints and tips for using contrast are provided throughout this book, including special sections in Chapter 7 Cooking and Eating, Chapter 8 Organize your Living Space, and Chapter 9 Find Hard-to-Spot Things. Many of the suggestions also involve the sense of touch. For tips on computer keyboards and monitors, see Chapter 13 Embrace Technology.

I discovered something new when I started this book's new edition. For easier reading on my computer monitor, I changed the color setting to white on black. When I switched back to black on white, the glare was so overpowering that I realized how much easier on my eyes it is to read white on black.

This option is available in Accessibility Preferences and is called "Invert colors." I wrote this entire book using the white on black option.

4

Read to Expand Horizons

TRADITIONAL, ELECTRONIC, AND AUDIO methods for reading printed material include audio technology for listening to recorded books; the use of low tech magnifiers, and, finally, electronic devices—high tech magnifiers, desktop computer programs that read text aloud, and electronic formats for reading on tablet computers and ebook readers.

Reading stands position hard copy

Rather than laying a book or newspaper flat on a table, or holding it upright with your hands, consider a reading stand—a handy way to maintain the best height and angle. If you usually need to move material to the left or right to match a "good spot" in your eye, a reading stand helps by keeping the reading material stationary, allowing you to move or tilt your head as needed. This may be easier than moving around books or papers.

The stand in the photo can be set at four different angles and three different heights. It holds all types of reading material, from a small book to an

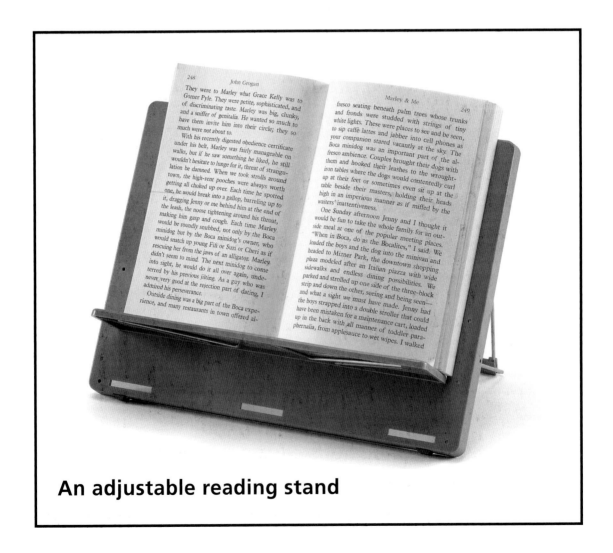

An adjustable reading stand

oversized atlas to a 5"-wide, triple-thick three-ring binder. It is especially good for propping up a newspaper. The use of a stand reduces arm and neck fatigue and promotes erect posture, encouraging the proper body alignment required for good balance. Other styles of reading stands are sometimes called copy holders, book holders, or book stands. Check low vision catalogs for a good selection.

Magnifying glasses

Magnifying glasses can enlarge print to be more readable. They are available at several magnification levels, from the lowest level, 2x, up to 15x. Try different magnification levels, starting with the lowest, until you find one that works for you. Do not "buy ahead" in case you need stronger magnification later on. Use the correct strength for your current vision. Go with the minimum magnification level required, because the higher the level, the smaller the view. You see fewer letters and words as the magnification increases, even when the dimensions of the magnifier remain consistent. If your doctor has given you a prescription, you will know what magnification level to order. If there is a low vision store in your area, you can experiment to find the magnification level that is right for you.

Magnifying glasses come in various shapes, sizes, and styles. One unusual style, called a pendant, features a rectangular or round magnifier that hangs around the neck on a cord or chain, keeping the magnifier handy. Other types include pocket magnifiers, cell phone magnifiers, and magnifying mirrors.

Illuminated magnifiers

Magnifying glasses are also available with battery-operated lights that illuminate the reading material. These are especially useful in low-light conditions and for people requiring more light to read. Low-priced illuminated magnifiers with LED lights come in powers ranging from 2x to 15x. Tabletop and floor lamps with magnifier arms are also available, as shown on page 36.

If greater magnification is required than is provided by magnifying glasses, consider trying one of the magnification systems that incorporates advanced technology. See description in Chapter 13.

Binoculars that attach to glasses

There are several types of binoculars that attach to eyeglasses or to a visor. Sports spectacles have the binoculars attached to a frame. These products are good for watching sporting events, TV, movies, and other distance viewing tasks. Consult low vision catalogs to view choices.

Listening to Books

The first recorded books were offered in 1931 by the passage of the Pratt-Smoot Act that established the Talking Book program of the National Library Service for the Blind and Physically Handicapped (NLS), administered by the Library of Congress.

The slogan of the NLS is "That All May Read." This free program loans recorded and Braille books and magazines in a number of languages, music scores in Braille and in large print, and specially designed playback equipment. Enrollment is open to those who are unable to read or use standard print materials due to visual or physical impairment. Through a national network of cooperating regional libraries, material is delivered free of charge right to your home by the

US Postal Service. Returns are also free, picked up at your mailbox.

The first playback machines used recorded discs. Audiocassette tapes were first available in 1969. New models of cassette playback machines were developed over the years, and in 1990 the first talking book machine with variable speed control was produced. This analog system became obsolete by the early 2000s, and the move to digital technology began.

In 2008 the Talking Book program transitioned to a digital flash memory system that uses a cartridge with a small playback machine that is much lighter than the cassette player. Books then became available both on cartridges and by download from the BARD (Braille and Audio Reading Download) website of the NLS. Features of the cartridge format include:

- speed control.

- tone control of voice.

- large storage capacity. One cartridge can hold multiple books.

Player is small and light—6" × 9" × 2" and slightly over two pounds.

Enrolling in the Talking Book program

US residents and citizens living abroad who meet one of the following criteria are eligible to participate in the Talking Book program.

- Persons whose visual disability, with correction, is certified by a competent authority as preventing the reading of standard printed material

- Persons certified by competent authority as unable to read or unable to use standard printed material as a result of physical limitations

- Persons certified by a competent authority as having a reading disability

- A competent authority can be ophthalmologists, optometrists, registered nurses, therapists, and hospital social workers, caseworkers, counselors, and rehabilitation teachers. In the absence of any of the above, ask a professional librarian.

How the program works

Once you are enrolled, you receive a playback machine from the regional center that provides the players. You start receiving the free publication *Talking Book Topics,* which is published every two months and available in large print, on audiocassette, and on the NLS website, www.loc.gov/nls/. The annotated list in each issue is limited to titles recently added to the national collection, which contains thousands of fiction and nonfiction titles, including classics, biographies, Gothics, mysteries, and how-to and self-help guides. There are special sections for children's and foreign language books. To learn more about the books in the national collection, readers can order catalogs and bibliographies by subject from cooperating libraries. Librarians can check other resources for titles and answer requests about special materials. There is online access to the complete library catalog via the NLS. You can search the complete collection by keyword, title, and author by going to www.loc.gov/nls/ and clicking on "Search the Catalog" at the top right of the home page.

—————— MY STORY ——————

Reading to Uncle Matt

When my Uncle Matt lost his central vision over fifty years ago, he was a practicing tax attorney who lived in St. Paul, Minnesota. He took the streetcar, by himself with his white cane, to the neighboring city of

Minneapolis to learn Braille at what was then called the Minneapolis Society for the Blind (now known as Vision Loss Resources). After class, he sometimes took the streetcar to our house in Minneapolis, where he spread out his large Braille sheets on the dining room table and proudly demonstrated how he could read. Before long he became a volunteer lawyer at a legal aid society.

Uncle Matt's hobby and great interest was the Civil War, and he missed being able to read new books published on the subject. Back then, there were a few Talking Book recordings on 33⅓ rpm records, but the program didn't offer recorded books on relatively specialized topics such as the Civil War. (By 2010 the National Library Service holdings online catalog listed 1,617 entries for the Civil War.) To help fill the Civil War void in my uncle's life, my husband-to-be and I made weekly trips to his house, where we took turns reading aloud the new books my uncle could no longer see.

Thirty years later, my mother, in her late seventies, learned she had macular degeneration after the cataract surgery that she'd expected would restore her vision made no improvement. Always an avid reader, her life began to revolve around Talking Books. I visited her every Wednesday, and my main activity was reading aloud the list of new books available and writing down the order for her selections. I kept a log of these selections in a notebook that I still have. Her cassette playback machine was awkward, the sound was poor, and she had to pass over many books she wanted to hear because she couldn't understand many high-pitched female voices. She found it difficult, while listening to a book, to keep track of the many cassette tapes required for most books. Still, with her life enhanced by her beloved Talking Books, my mother enjoyed a life of spirited acceptance until she died at the age of eighty-eight.

Now, twenty-five years later, I still look forward to the day when I can catch up on all the reading I have not yet been able to fit into my life. But I will not be waiting for a visitor to read to me or struggle with cassettes and their playback machine. Instead I will listen to books on a lightweight device or, more likely, download books from the Talking Book Internet site. This is an exciting and comforting prospect for me.

Commercial sources of recorded books—CDs and ebooks

In addition to the NLS books you can borrow for free with delivery to your home, books are available for purchase in various formats.

- Audiobooks on compact discs for CD players are available for purchase at "brick-and-mortar" bookstores and on a multitude of websites. You listen to these books on a regular CD player. List prices range from $20.00 up, but they are often sold at discounted prices. They are also available for loan from public libraries. Audio books in MP3 formats can be downloaded from websites onto computers or MP3 players.

- Ebooks for digital reading devices

An ebook is an electronic version of a printed book that is available for download from the Internet. Ebooks can be read on electronic devices—ebook readers that are dedicated to books and tablet computers that also provide access to email and the Internet, including magazines and newspapers, plus all the information available on Internet websites.

The devices offer several useful options—

- Text size is adjustable.
- Multiple fonts are available.
- Page orientation can be horizontal or vertical.
- Text reflows to fill the available view area.
- Large capacity can hold a huge number of books.

There are several brands, and each has its own format. Choose one with a large screen and a non-serif (sans serif) font that is easy to read.

5

Nurture Your Body

BENEFIT YOUR EYES with a healthy diet and exercise. Our body fitness is interconnected with our minds. This connection can bolster our resilience and help us develop new skills to maintain a fulfilling and independent life.

Guidelines for a healthy lifestyle

Many factors contribute to physical well-being. Eyes, like any other part of the body, benefit from a healthful diet. Suggested guidelines for a healthy lifestyle from the National Eye Institute of the US National Institutes of Health, and from retinologists, are listed here. The recommendations are important for everyone, but particularly important for anyone with an eye disease. Since there is often a genetic factor, the guidelines are also important for one's children and grandchildren. In my case, my mother, uncle, first cousin, and a second cousin all developed a macular disease, and we've traced it back to the maternal side of my mother's family. Your entire family would benefit from following these guidelines.

- Exercise and increase physical activity.

- Eat a healthful diet high in fruits, green leafy vegetables (especially kale and spinach for macular degeneration), and fish.

- Watch your weight and reduce your fat intake.

- Maintain normal blood pressure and cholesterol levels.

- Do not smoke.

- If you have diabetes, it is important to control your levels of blood sugar, blood pressure, and blood cholesterol. Doing so can help prevent the development and progression of diabetic retinopathy.

Doctors recommend that your adult children have annual eye examinations, even if they do not require eyeglasses, starting at age fifty; and at the appointment, tell the doctor about the family history of macular disease.

Balance and body awareness

In addition to the five commonly known senses (sight, hearing, taste, touch, and smell), two other senses are especially important for people with vision loss. The first is the perception of balance. The second is the perception of your own body—the awareness of your posture and positioning and feelings of movements of your body. We rely on looking ahead at objects to anchor ourselves in the space we occupy. These are senses that people are frequently not aware of, but rely on enormously even, if unconsciously.

Exercise for independence

During exercise, the brain and muscles learn to communicate more efficiently and help us build confidence in the way our bodies move. Being active helps ensure that you can maintain independence with regard to the activities of daily living, such as grooming, bathing, dressing, preparing food, and walking.

Motivating yourself to exercise can be difficult, but physical activity is crucial to nurturing your body. You do not need to excel at sports to gain from and enjoy exercise, and you can start at any age and still receive great benefits. Before starting an exercise program, make an appointment with your doctor, who may offer suggestions on specific types of exercise from among the types listed below.

- Aerobic exercise to improve cardiovascular fitness, immune function, cognitive function, and mood

- Strength training to build and maintain muscle and bone mass

- Flexibility training to improve motion throughout each body joint

- Balance training to prevent falls and develop confident movement

Although each type of exercise is important, balance training is especially critical for someone with vision loss. Falling is a very real danger when it is difficult to see your surroundings. Follow the suggestions below when developing your general fitness program.

- Consult health professionals, such as physical and occupational therapists, for a determination of your strengths and areas of deficit.

- Add their recommendations for balance training to your exercise program.

- Work to develop a good internal sense of balance and the ability to quickly right yourself when thrown off balance.

- Wear shoes with good fit and support. Choose soles that prevent slipping but do not excessively grip the floor, which can lead to injury if your foot doesn't follow the turn of your body.

- Take extra care when you are tired, stressed, or distracted, so you can respond as needed to challenges.

- Adequate rest helps to ensure quick responses by body and mind.

- Learn exercises and do them in ten-minute periods throughout the day—you'll benefit just as much from these short separate sessions as you would from one long session.

Find a fitness class

After consulting a healthcare professional, consider joining a fitness class to stay motivated and receive instruction on how to properly perform exercises. Classes are offered in community recreation centers, community education programs, senior centers, churches, and low vision organizations. If you join or belong to a health club or gym, you can have individual instruction from a trainer who can design a program for you.

You might find it helpful to attend classes in yoga, Pilates, and/or Tai Chi. Tai Chi is especially helpful because it helps to develop inner balance without relying on focusing on a spot in the distance, which you may already be doing to anchor yourself when doing balance exercises. Choosing physical activities that you enjoy encourages you to practice consistently at home to gain optimal benefits.

If you are not physically able to take a class or do standing exercises at home, you can do chair exercises sitting in your own living room. Most states have a service that provides a closed-circuit radio network with special programming for those unable to read or hold reading material. An exercise program is often included in the service's scheduled programming.

My mother regularly did chair exercises even though she had severe arthritis and only peripheral vision. These sessions helped her keep a positive attitude and seemed to make her feel better. You can find a radio station in your area by checking the International Association of Audio Information Services website at www.iaaais.org/locateservice.html or by calling your state's department of services for the blind. You can also listen to broadcasts of these radio programs on the Internet. See page 222–223 for more information on these radio services. Also, public and community television stations sometimes offer exercise programming.

Strength and agility for driving

Another motivation to exercise is to be able to keep driving as long as possible. Some people mistakenly believe that good vision is all that is required for driving. If you stop to think about all the muscle groups you use to drive, you can understand how exercise can help keep you behind the wheel.

You must have agility to be a safe driver. Just to climb into the car, you need strong leg and upper body muscles. Your foot, ankle, and calf muscles must be strong and flexible for pushing the pedals to brake and accelerate. Your arms, wrists, and fingers are needed for steering and using dashboard controls. Your neck must be flexible and strong to be able to turn to check blind spots when changing lanes. Torso strength and agility are needed so that you can twist to the left and right to see what is behind you when preparing to back up. Driving is definitely a full-body activity.

See Chapter 10 for a more detailed discussion of driving.

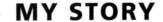 **MY STORY**

Athletic Failure, But Exercise Lover

As a child, teenager, and college student, I tried one sport after the other, both in gym classes and at neighborhood ball games. Whether it was softball, basketball, volleyball, swimming, or, finally, golf— I was the last person wanted on any team. I totally lacked whatever it is that makes one able to perform at even a minimum level in sports.

Then, in my early twenties, I discovered an adult beginners' ballet class and found the joy of dance. Although not innately talented, I was able to do the classic exercises at the barre, and I advanced to work in the center of the room where there was nothing to hold on to. I continued classes for a few years, then stopped until my late forties, when I found another adult beginners' class. My love of balletic exercise was renewed, and I took classes for another couple of years.

Thirty years passed until I found a ballet class for mature adults offered through my community's adult education program. By then I was seventy-four years old, and my body had forgotten everything it had once known about ballet. My teachers, a husband-and-wife team, were tolerant, and they welcomed me into their beginning and intermediate classes.

Through another lucky connection, I discovered Pilates, a mind-body exercise system with an approach to movement that emphasizes body alignment, breathing, strength, flexibility, balance, and endurance. My instructor, who is also an occupational therapist, knew exactly how to help me develop the strength and balance to move forward with my study of ballet.

I was still missing strength and aerobic training components, and at the age of eighty, I added kettlebells (cast-iron weights that look like bowling balls with a handle on top) to my program. These exercise activities bring me a feeling of exhilaration, and they have given me a level of fitness that has helped me through some trying times. I need the sustenance of body and spirit that exercise provides. This has helped to develop the resilience to bounce back and deal with new challenges in my life.

———————————

Personal care

Try the ideas below as you go about your personal care tasks.

Talking healthcare products

A huge variety of specialty products provide audio as well as visual information to help you take care of personal healthcare tasks. They are available at low vision stores. Here are some "talking" products.

- Blood pressure monitors

- Glucose meters

- Pedometers that announce the numbers of steps you have taken and total distance traveled

- Scales that speak your weight or with detachable displays that you can hold as close to your eyes as needed to read them

- Thermometers that state your temperature reading

Brushing teeth

- An electric toothbrush that is kept upright in a charger on your vanity or counter is easy to find.

- Toothpaste in a pump dispenser that stands upright on the counter is easier to find than a tube that is harder to see when laying on your bathroom vanity.

- Match up the toothpaste from the dispenser with the toothbrush bristles by first putting the toothpaste on your finger, then transferring it to the toothbrush. Even easier, put toothpaste on your finger, then transfer it directly to your mouth.

- I learned a good trick when friends in ballet class and other places told me I had toothpaste around my mouth and even on my cheek. I can no longer see in the mirror well enough to know that I'm not "smeared." Now I always splash water all over my face, or even better, wipe with a wet washcloth.

Have a spot-finder buddy

If you live with someone, make an agreement that he or she will always tell you when you have a spot on your clothing or face—toothpaste around your mouth, lipstick on your teeth, or shaving cream under your ear. This will be a great service to you, as spots can be almost impossible to see. A buddy system with a housemate or friend can prevent you from going around with embarrassing spots, unbeknownst to you.

Grooming

- Lipstick can end up in the wrong spot, such as on your teeth or "outside the lines." Instead, try tinted lip gloss which is not as noticeable when you mis-aim. Lip gloss usually costs less than lipstick, and many also act as a moisturizing lip balm.

- Close your eyes when using hair spray or applying makeup with a brush to avoid getting in your eyes.

- Magnifying mirrors for close-work grooming tasks are available in many sizes, shapes, and magnification levels. Some are lighted. Some models are handheld, on stands, or wall-mounted with the magnifiers at the end of swivel arms.

- Use an electric razor for shaving safety.

Bathing and showering

- Installing grabs bars in your tub and shower will help you stay oriented and provide a means of support when getting in and out.

- Use a shower bench or transfer bench if you are unsteady in the shower or find it difficult to enter or exit the tub or shower.

Caring for nails

- Use emery boards instead of nail clippers to keep fingernails and toenails trimmed. Filing by feel keeps you from accidentally cutting too much or injuring yourself.

- Have a regular pedicure if basic toenail care is difficult for you. Home visits by pedicurists or nurses are available in some communities, and from many senior centers. If you would rather not visit a pedicurist for basic toenail maintenance, but you have a hard time reaching your toes or seeing your nails, enlist the help of a friend or relative who can file your toenails with an emery board.

- Visit a podiatrist for nail clipping and to care for ingrown toenails or other foot-related problems, such as corns or calluses. Visits every two months are covered for those with Medicare.

Spots on clothing

Spray with spot remover or wash out a spot on clothing right away. If that doesn't work, as an extra precaution, mark the spot with a safety pin and pre-treat the area before placing the garment in the washer. For items that must be dry cleaned, safety pins identify areas that require special treatment.

Laundry detergent packets

Premeasured dissolvable packets, rather than powder or liquid detergent, solve the problem of measuring the right amount of laundry detergent for your washer. Several brands are also available for dishwashers.

AFB report on washers and dryers

AccessWorld News, published by the American Federation of the Blind (AFB), reports the results of its research on the accessibility of appliances, along with other product categories. Washers and dryers were reported on in the May 2007 issue. Check for a more recent report with the online search term: AFB washers. Washers have multiple settings and touch controls more often; so, if you need a new washer and dryer, check to see if you can find models that still use knobs.

Matching socks

Even people with good vision can find it difficult to pair up socks as they come out of the dryer. Here are two tricks to make this a snap.

- To eliminate the problem, have all identical socks—one style, one color—so that no matching is needed. Once you find a style you like, buy multiple pairs, and you won't have to worry about matching up socks again.

- If you prefer a variety of socks, use large safety pins to fasten pairs together at the toe or heel when you take them off. Color code socks by using two or more pins for colors other than black or white. If you do laundry for others, be sure that they follow this system as well.

Ironing

The best way to avoid ironing is to wear wrinkle-free clothes. But if you do need to iron, follow these safety precautions.

- Use a paint pen to place high marks on the iron settings.

- Place the ironing board next to a heatproof kitchen counter.

- Put the iron on the counter, not on the ironing board, while you prepare to iron or need to set the iron down to rearrange an item.

- Pour water into the iron through a funnel.

- Never grope around trying to find a hot iron. Instead, lightly run your hand along the cord to find it. As your hand gets close to the iron, you should be able to feel its heat. Stop before you accidentally touch the hot face of the iron.

- Use your hands to find wrinkles to smooth.

6

Develop Your Senses of Touch and Hearing

COMPENSATE WITH TOUCH AND HEARING as your sense of sight diminishes. Start thinking about your sense of touch, which you may have taken for granted. You will identify things by feel that you formerly could see. We feel through nerve endings that act as touch receptors through our skin. Our fingertips are especially sensitive, because they have more receptors than most other parts of the body. Just think about how much a small paper cut on the tip of your finger hurts. This sensitivity allows you to feel the difference between rough and smooth, soft and hard, hot and cold, and wet and dry. Feeling an object tells you if it is flat or raised, round or square. Later chapters describe how your sense of touch is important in the kitchen and in finding hard-to-spot things that have been identified with special marks.

Find pleasure in textures

Some items that give sensory pleasure when touched or stroked include fabrics such as fleece or velvet, rocks and pebbles, smooth or textured glass, and wood or metal objects and sculpture. Petting your cat or dog gives pleasure to both you and your pet. Hugs are felt through your skin. Hugs can reduce stress and make you feel good all over. Look for things you enjoy feeling and touching, to enjoy now—and later.

Identify objects by feel

As you go about your daily activities, pay attention to the shapes and sizes of objects you use throughout the day. When you put away dishes, for instance, you can tell the difference between large and small plates and bowls and short and tall glasses. This enables you to put things in their designated places in your cupboards, even when it's difficult to see where they belong. Learn to tell the difference between knives, forks, and spoons by their shapes and weights. I remember watching my mother and her blind brother, my Uncle Matt, put away silverware after the feast at family celebrations. I can still hear her saying, "You can tell the good silverware by its heft and weight. Keep it separate from the everyday knives and forks."

Sense of touch in the kitchen is covered further in the next chapter.

Identifying money

Finding the correct amount of money in your wallet or coin purse is another new skill that involves the sense of touch. My Uncle Matt showed me a system of keeping track of paper currency fifty years ago. It fascinated me then, and it is still in use today. He folded each denomination of paper money in a different way.

- One dollar: unfolded

- Five dollars: folded in half crosswise

- Ten dollars: folded in quarters

- Twenty dollars: folded in half lengthwise

If you don't like his system, develop your own, or use one of these ideas:

- Put each denomination in a different pocket in your purse.

- Secure five-dollar bills with a small paper clip and ten-dollar bills with a large paper clip. Use no clips for one-dollar bills.

Coins can be identified by paying attention to their sizes and feel. Tell the difference between a quarter and a dime or penny by the coins' sizes is easy, but what about distinguishing quarters from nickels, or pennies from dimes? Feel for ridges on the rims of the coins. Quarters and dimes have ridges you can feel, making them distinguishable from nickels and pennies.

Money organizer wallets designed especially for the visually impaired feature four separate compartments for one, five, ten and twenty dollar bills, plus three separate change purses. There are multiple slots for credit cards, plus an extra compartment to hold miscellaneous items like charge slips. These wallets are available from low vision stores.

Optimize your sense of hearing

As sight diminishes, hearing becomes more and more important. We may not realize how frequently we use our hearing in many areas of our lives, such as when driving—a strong motivation to have your hearing tested if you suspect a hearing loss. As your sight diminishes, good hearing helps you maintain connections with other people.

Develop your listening skills

I learned the importance of listening from four panelists with Stargardt disease who spoke at a Foundation Fighting Blindness chapter meeting. They ranged in age from twelve to sixty-two, but all emphasized the importance of listening. I was impressed that they all identify people by their voices. One mentioned listening to the emotion in speakers' voices because she can't see facial expressions. Others attend audio-described plays. I want to develop my own skills for listening to audio books when I can no longer read large print. I will also be listening to the computer speaking what is on the screen. Now I ask questions and receive spoken replies from the assistant on my smart phone.

Have your hearing checked

Have your hearing checked by a licensed audiologist to ensure that you receive a thorough examination. If you go to an ear doctor for an examination, the doctor can probably refer you to an audiologist if you need a hearing aid. Simply responding to an ad you receive in the mail for a "free hearing evaluation" may not result in the comprehensive evaluation you require, and you may be shown only one brand of hearing aid, which may not be the best for you. Medicare covers the costs of hearing tests, so you can have your hearing tested by a reputable, licensed audiologist. Entrust your hearing only to a qualified professional.

Licensed audiologists may work in private practices or in hospitals or clinics. If there are underlying medical issues causing your hearing to be affected, your audiologist may refer you to an ENT (ear, nose, and throat) physician, also called an otolaryngologist. If hearing tests show that you would be helped by a hearing aid, the audiologist can discuss a variety of hearing aid choices with you.

If you have a hearing loss, you will greatly benefit from using hearing aids. Unfortunately, they can be expensive and are not covered by Medicare. Some health insurance plans pay a portion of the cost, but not every year. If the price is out of your reach, discuss your situation with your audiologist—sometimes arrangements can be made for a manufacturer or other source to help with the expense.

Hearing aid batteries

Use of a hearing aid involves the sense of touch. It requires good finger dexterity to insert a hearing aid in your ear. Although removal is easier, dexterity is still required. It is quite possible to accidentally drop an aid on the floor. A bigger challenge is handling the batteries.

My first two hearing aids were "completely in the canal" models that used number-10 batteries. I got the first aid, for my left ear, in 1996—long before I had any vision loss. Handling the tiny batteries was no problem until my vision decreased, and I could barely see where to insert a new battery. I tried changing a battery with my eyes closed, but was not successful. Even with my eyes open, I was dropping the tiny batteries on the floor. Eventually I learned to change batteries over a counter or table to minimize the danger of them falling. Sitting in an upholstered chair to change a battery can lead to the battery falling into a cranny of the chair, making it even harder to find than one that has landed on the floor.

Dropped or lost batteries can be more than aggravating to find—and they can be dangerous to a pet or a young child who might be attracted to them and swallow them. Even though hearing aid batteries no longer contain mercury and do not need to be recycled, they can cause serious gastric problems if swallowed.

I now have large, behind-the-ear hearing aids for both ears. They use the large, number-13 battery. My audiologist picked out the brand of aid that was

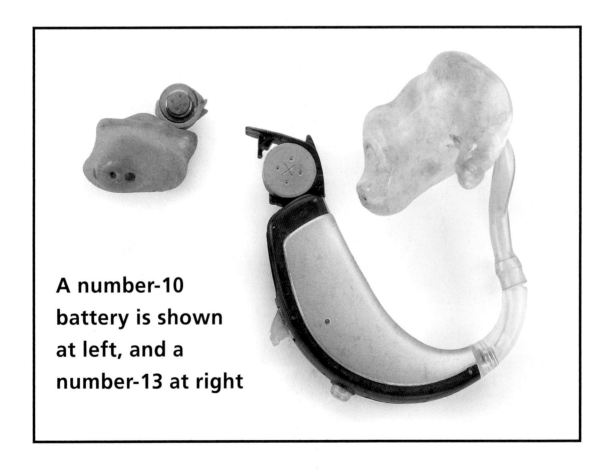

A number-10 battery is shown at left, and a number-13 at right

easiest in terms of changing batteries. I practiced changing the battery with my eyes closed several times, and I was successful.

When I began using the first aid with the number-13 battery, my hearing was still at a level that would have allowed me to continue using another small hearing aid that required number-10 batteries. But I wanted to be prepared for both future hearing loss and the need to manipulate the batteries with diminished vision. My aids are currently set a little above the middle volume level, and the audiologist can program the volume to higher levels as needed.

Are you lip reading?

I was surprised when my audiologist had me take tests that showed that I was relying heavily on lip reading, without even realizing it. First she placed me in a booth with a glass wall dividing us. I was wearing earphones that allowed me to hear her voice, and I could see her on the other side of the glass wall as she read word after word. As she said each word, I tried to repeat it back to her. She kept a score of how many I got correct. Then I closed my eyes so that I could not see her enunciating the words. I was amazed to learn that I got 92 percent of the words correct when I was watching the audiologist, but only 72 percent correct when I could not see her. These results showed that I was doing a lot of lip reading.

These helpful strategies for dealing with a hearing loss, when you also have diminished vision, were suggested to me by my audiologist.

- Train yourself to listen—try closing your eyes when watching television or chatting with someone, or listen to an audio book.

- Ask people to speak slowly and enunciate clearly.

- Ask people to look directly at you when speaking so that the sound comes directly to you. Even if you can't watch their lips, you may be able to see their body language and gestures, such as arm waving— valuable cues that help you understand what the speakers are saying.

- Find the best listening spot in your house of worship by trying different seating locations.

- Use assistive listening devices at movies, theaters, concerts, and other such venues.

- In restaurants, ask for a quiet table off to the side, near a wall. Face the wall rather than the room—if you sit facing the room, with the noise in front of you and a wall behind you, the speaker's voice at your table can become overpowered by the other noise coming right at you from the room. When you face the wall, the loudest sounds come from the people speaking at your table who are facing you. The texture of the wall behind you can make a difference in whether more sound reflects off of it as well.

Most important of all—be an advocate for yourself, and let others know what you need.

MY STORY

The Dog Ate My Hearing Aid

Be careful where you put your hearing aids. Even more dangerous to a pet than swallowing a battery is eating an entire hearing aid. If you have a pet, place your aids in their containers when you remove them from your ears. Dogs and cats are attracted to the hum of a hearing aid that hasn't been turned off, as well as to the scent of wax that may adhere to the inner part of a hearing aid.

When I still had the small aid, I carelessly placed my aid on my bedside table before an afternoon rest. That night, my son's dog became violently ill. I didn't make the connection until a couple of days later when I realized my aid was hopelessly lost. Fortunately the hearing aid was very small and the dog recovered, but a larger aid could have caused serious internal injuries. Things turned out just fine for the dog, but I had to spend hundreds of dollars on a new hearing aid.

———————————

Cooking and Eating

GOOD DIET AND NUTRITION are essential parts of a healthy lifestyle, and food preparation is an important activity of daily life. The ideas in this chapter will help you cook and eat without assistance from others. Can you guess which sense other than sight is most important when cooking? You might first think of taste, then smell. You may be surprised by how important your sense of touch is in compensating for a diminishing sense of sight. Hearing also becomes important in the kitchen.

As you go about your tasks in the kitchen, be aware of activities that are becoming difficult, and start thinking about new ways to do them. Be creative in finding solutions to cooking challenges. Use the ideas here to get you started. Some are my own and some I learned in an inspiring "Independent Living Skills" class I took at Vision Loss Resources in Minneapolis. The methods taught were gathered from participants who shared their ideas over thirty years.

Useful items in the kitchen

Use these items as you learn new ways to cook

- Set of metal measuring cups with raised dots (See pages 88–89)
- Saucer
- Funnels of various sizes
- Needle-nose pliers or ring opener
- Timer with large numbers that talks or has loud ring
- Towels—one dark, one light
- Cutting boards—one dark, one light—or various colors
- Heavy rubber bands
- Pair of insulated gloves with nonslip silicone grips

Contrast makes cooking and eating easier

These tips can make meal preparation and eating less frustrating and more enjoyable.

- To brighten and make it easier find items in kitchen cupboards, place white shelf liner on the shelves—top, bottom, and sides.

- To catch spills when mixing ingredients, place a dark towel underneath a white bowl; place a white towel under a dark bowl.

- To measure dark-colored foods like coffee, use white measuring cups and spoons; to measure light-colored foods like flour and sugar, use dark measuring cups and spoons.

- To slice light foods, such as onions, use a dark-colored cutting board; use a light-colored cutting board to slice dark foods, such as cooked meat.

- To better see when to stop pouring a dark liquid such as coffee, use a cup that's light on the inside. A cup with a dark rim at the top is even better.

- For white liquids, use a colored glass or one with a pattern. Water can be difficult to see in any type of glass because it is transparent.

- Use colored or patterned drinking glasses rather than transparent glasses because they are easier to see and to avoid knocking over.

- Avoid plates with patterns, which can be visually confusing when you are trying to locate your food.
- Use different colored dishes, depending on the color of the foods served.

Use sense of touch in the kitchen

If you have difficulty identifying items such as measuring cups and spoons or dials on the stove and oven, a solution is to use a special paint pen to apply small dots of paint that raise, harden, and become waterproof and dishwasher-proof. These dots are informally known as "high marks." You can develop your sense of touch by feeling the number of dots on the handles and dials on your appliances.

Paint pens are available at low vision stores. They come in a variety of colors, including black, white, and orange. The paint adheres to just about any surface, including plastic and metal. One brand of tactile paint pen is the HI-MARK™. The dots are produced by squirting a paint-like substance from the pen onto the surface you want to mark.

In order to make sure there is plenty of space for placing the dots, use metal measuring cups and

Apply a dot using a HI-MARK™ pen.

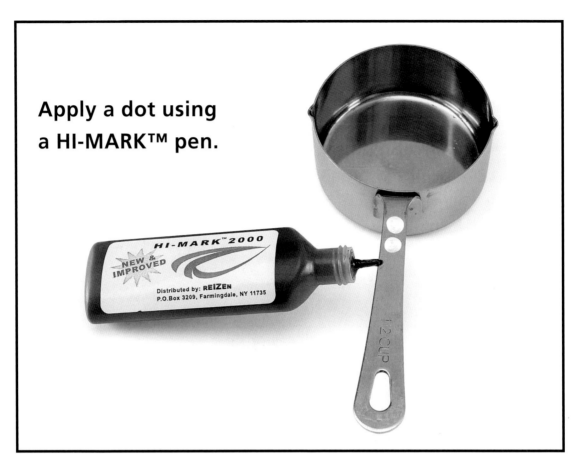

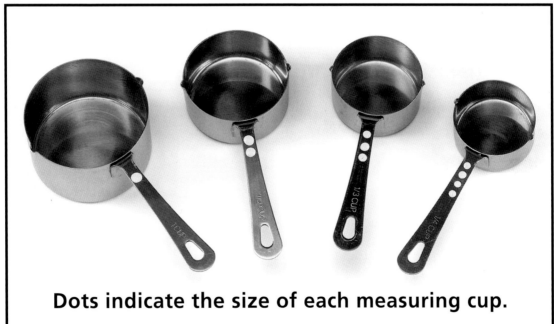

Dots indicate the size of each measuring cup.

spoons with long handles. Place the dots on the handles close to the cup or spoon, so you are able to grasp the handles and slide your thumb along the top of the handle to feel the number of dots. To tell one measuring cup from another, put one dot on the 1-cup measure, two dots on the ½-cup measure, three dots on the ⅓-cup measure, and four dots on the ¼-cup measure. Use a similar system with measuring spoons.

Selecting kitchen appliances

Technology keeps changing on stoves, wall ovens, cooktops, microwaves, dishwashers, as well as washers and dryers. Older appliances are often easier to use, because the controls of newer models are not as accessible for those with low vision. Most newer electric and gas stoves have a combination of touch pads for the oven and knobs for the burners. The oven control is often placed on the rear splashguard, making it more difficult to reach or see. Traditional coiled electric burners are sometimes concealed below smooth ceramic cooktops, making it difficult to see where to place the pan.

When visiting major retailers in 2013 I found only one stove with traditional knob controls for burners and oven. It was the cheapest on the floor. Low-end basic models with traditional controls may not be on the showroom floor, so inquire about what might be available by special order.

Microwave cooking

Use your sense of hearing: listen closely to the number of beeps when you press the buttons to set the cooking time. One extra push of the minute button, for instance, could lead to overcooking, a smoke-filled oven, or worse.

When selecting a new microwave oven, look for a model with some of the following special options.

- A "30 seconds" button, so you can easily set the time for ½, 1½, or 2½ minutes.

- A "talking" feature that can prompt you to set the time and announce cooking time settings, the running cooking time, the current power level, and such phrases as "microwave running," "attend to food," and so forth. High-end models that announce the current time and have a speech volume control are available at low vision stores.

- A sensor helps to prevent overcooking or undercooking by determining when the food is ready based on infrared light or by the steam emitted from the food.

- Choose the door handle that works best for you, whether it requires pulling or has a bar or button to push to open the door.

Dishwasher detergent packets

Dishwashers have touchpad controls with many settings. To identify your normal setting, place a raised plastic bump on both that and the start touchpad. For detergent, premeasured, dissolvable packets (rather than loose powder, liquids, or gels) solve the problem of getting the right amount into the small container in the dishwasher. As with laundry detergent, there are several brands.

Large print and specialty cookbooks

Many cookbooks are available in large print versions. You can find the books in many libraries and some bookstores. Online booksellers, such as Amazon (www.amazon.com) and Large Print Books (www.largeprintbooks.com), carry a wide variety of large print titles.

If you have a medical condition that restricts your diet, nutrition becomes even more important. Take the time and effort to find foods you enjoy. Consult a specialty cookbook, available for diabetic, cardiac, renal, and gluten-free diets. In fact, no matter what dietary restrictions you have, there is probably at least one cookbook that will work for you, and some come in large print editions.

Using recipes

Because you will use your fingers in new ways, always start by washing your hands. Place a towel on your work space for contrast, to catch drips and spills, and to keep bowls and cutting boards from sliding. When making something in a mixing bowl, first lay out all your ingredients to one side of the bowl. After each ingredient is added, move its container to the other side of the bowl. Then you do not have to wonder whether you have added a particular item.

Measuring ingredients

Your sense of touch again comes into play when using measuring cups and spoons. If you are working with wet ingredients, keep a saucer handy as a place to put measuring cups and spoons that may drip. When measuring dry ingredients such as flour or sugar, select the size of measure you want and dip it into the canister. Rather than using a knife to level the scoopful—your index finger is a much "handier" instrument!

For small amounts of wet and liquid ingredients, use measuring spoons that are bent to form dippers. If you cannot see how much of an ingredient is in a measuring spoon, use your finger to "feel off" the top.

Using a knife on a cutting board

The safe way to find the sharp side of a knife is by touch. Grasp the handle and use your index finger to feel the notch at the end. The side with the notch is the sharp side, so turn the knife so that side is on the bottom. Silicone cutting boards come in a variety of bright colors to assist with contrast.

Cooking on a range or stovetop

Use your other senses to prepare food on stovetops.

- Rolling boils can be detected in two ways—by hearing the boil, or by placing your hand a few inches above the pan to feel the amount of steam being produced.

- Judge whether or not onions have become golden brown by sampling some that have cooled a bit. The taste of the onion and its tender texture lets you know.

- When frying foods, place a splatter guard on top of the pan. The guard prevents hot grease and little pieces of food from flying out of the pan to those hard-to-spot, hard-to-clean places on your stove.

Electric skillet for safety

If you feel unsafe using a frying pan on the stove, buy an electric skillet. The model I have has a separate heat control that plugs into the skillet. The control has a dial similar to that of an oven's temperature heat-setting dial, but with a top temperature of 400 degrees.

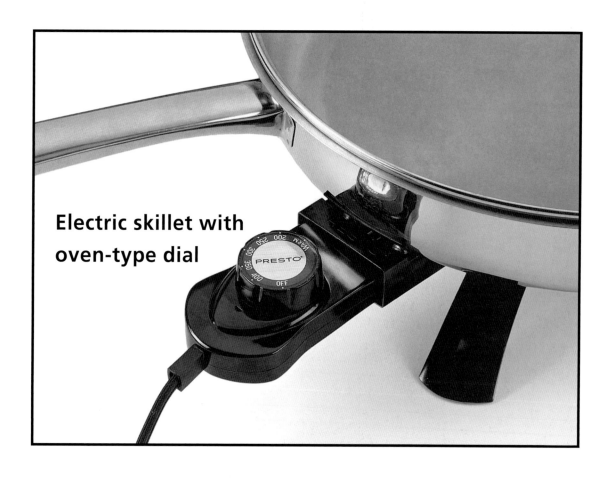

Electric skillet with oven-type dial

Insulated gloves for safety

Never reach into a hot or heating oven to place a pan on the rack or to remove the pan from the rack. Instead, always wear your insulated gloves to pull out the rack and place or remove your pan. This safety measure prevents burns, and should also be followed when cooking on the stove top. I learned this lesson when frying and my pot holder caught fire from the gas flame. Disaster was narrowly averted by my quick action, but a burn remains on my countertop.

Using timers

Timers can alert you when it is time to check to see if food is ready. Many types and sizes are available from low vision stores. Timers range in size from small digital models that are about 3" in height to a dial model that is 9" in diameter and has a loud and long ring. My favorite kitchen timer is a white on black model that is 7" × 9" and has a loud, 15-second ring. You may want to try a few different types. Timers don't have to be used just for cooking—you

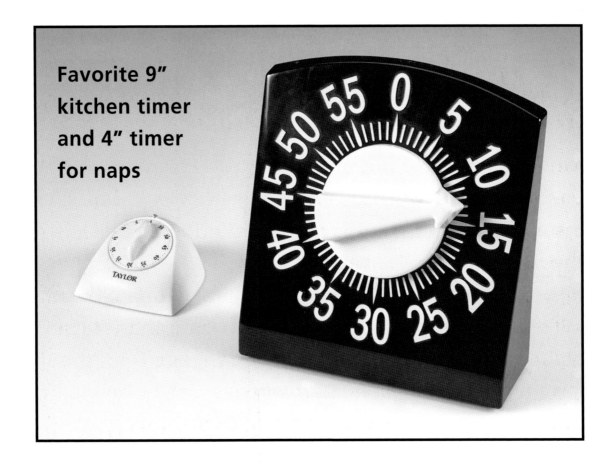

Favorite 9" kitchen timer and 4" timer for naps

may want to also keep some in other rooms, such as your bedroom to awaken you from a nap. Now I use dial-type timers because I am no longer able to read digital numbers.

Managing coffee-making

I enjoy a couple of cups of coffee when I get up in the morning, and have developed useful tricks to avoid several possible hazards. My first step was to get a 12" × 16" plastic tray with a lip all the way around. These are available at discount stores, and they come in a variety of bright colors. First place a towel on the tray, and then put all the items you need on the tray:

- Coffeemaker
- Coffee can
- Funnel
- Cups
- Straws

Follow these steps:

- Fill the carafe to the level for the number of cups you want. Place bumps (See pages 126–128 to learn about raised bumps) or paint the lines at the number of cups you usually make. See page 126 for instructions on using these markers.

Tray with coffee maker and funnel

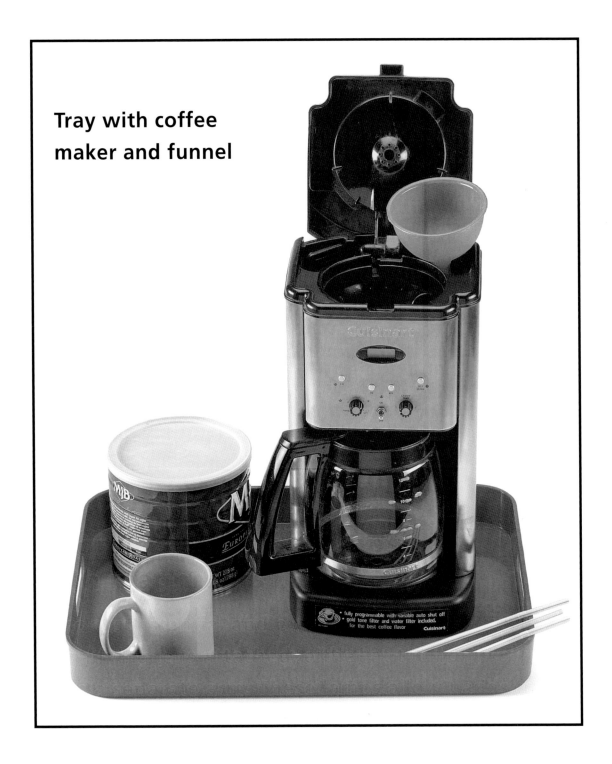

- Use a funnel when you can't see the hole for pouring the water into the coffeemaker, and slowly pour the water into the funnel—with no splashes or spills.

- Put the desired number of scoops into the basket. To check the level of coffee in the scoop, hold it with one hand and feel the top with your index finger, leveling off if necessary.

- When pouring my morning coffee, I place my cup on a small saucer so coffee doesn't get all over the counter when I pour over the top of the cup.

- If you pour over the top and coffee overflows, do not attempt to pick up the cup. Put a straw into the coffee cup and sip enough coffee to make it safe to pick up the cup.

- To see the cup on the dark table, I put my cup on a white paper napkin to make it visible. This is safer than a coaster that is raised above the table and easier to tip. I haven't broken a cup yet!

More tricks from low vision cooks

- Measure out one tablespoon from a stick of butter by using your index finger as a measure, placing it flat, perpendicular to the length of the butter.

- Canola oil (one of the more healthful oils) is the only oil that remains a liquid when stored in the refrigerator. When pouring it into a glass or cup, you are able to feel the level of the chilled liquid.

- Spray the inside of measuring cups with vegetable oil spray so food doesn't stick to the cups.

- Use oil sprays over the sink so you don't get any on the floor and slip.

- Marinate meat in a zipped plastic bag.

- Find which side of a milk carton to open by sliding your finger along the top to feel which side has the crease.

- To open cans with pull tabs, use needle-nose pliers or just stick a spoon under the tab.

- To reduce the amount of time you need to spend cooking, make multiple portions of favorite meals; and freeze individual servings for quick, handy meals that you can heat in the microwave oven.

Eating out

Eating at a restaurant need not be frustrating. Follow these tips, and enjoy your meal with confidence.

Restaurant seating

- Ask for a table or booth where the lighting is brightest.

- If you are troubled by glare, ask to be seated where glare is not present or where blinds can be drawn.

- If you are hard of hearing, ask for a table where the level of noise is low. See pages 82–83 for more tips where to sit in a restaurant when you have hearing loss.

Reading menus

- Bring a small flashlight to help you read the menu.

- An alternative is a magnifying glass with a light.

- If you are unable to read the menu, ask your dining companion to read it out loud for you—this can prompt some fun discussions.

- If you are dining alone and unable to read the menu, ask the server to read the sections, such as appetizers, main courses, or desserts that interest you.

- You can avoid the menu entirely by asking the server for the specials of the day or for personal recommendations.

- Decide on your selections before you leave home by checking the restaurant's website to look at the menu and decide what you are going to order.

Eating in low restaurant light

- Select finger food or easy-to-eat dishes that don't require cutting and are easy to distinguish on a plate.

- Ask that meat be cut in the kitchen.

- Laugh when you completely miss what you're aiming for with your fork and try to spear the table instead.

─────────────── **MY STORY** ───────────────

The Befuddled Servers

On the last evening of my visit with my daughter in Iowa City, we decided to have dinner at our favorite restaurant. It was a lovely August evening, so we decided to sit at an outdoor table. We already knew what we would splurge on: the tenderloin steak accompanied by a salad and vegetable. There were two servers, elegant in their long black aprons. I asked that my steak be cut in the kitchen because it was difficult for me to see due to my poor eyesight. And I was quite proud of myself for this bit of self-advocacy. I didn't want to spend our dinner struggling to cut my steak and then giving up and handing my plate over to my daughter.

Soon the two servers arrived and set our plates before us. By then, dusk was falling. I able to see that the large dark hunk on the far side of my plate had not been cut per my request.

In an exasperated voice, I exclaimed, "But, I asked that my steak be cut in the kitchen!"

The two servers looked at each other with bewildered expressions, then looked to my daughter for help. She said, "Mom, that's your salad!

I burst out laughing, followed by my daughter's laughter, and then the two servers'—who appeared relieved to know how to react.

_____

8

Organize Your Living Space

HAVE YOU ACCUMULATED all sorts of stuff over the years? If you have lived in the same place for a long time, it may be difficult to follow the common advice to sort through all those possessions and keep only what you really want and use. If you have recently downsized to a smaller place, this task won't be as hard as it is for someone like me, who continues to live in the same house since 1965.

In addition to organizing the things where you live, analyze your living quarters to make sure there are no safety hazards, such as obstacles you might not see. You can maximize the visibility of large objects, such as furniture. Some low vision organizations make home visits to check the safety of your home and offer help in making it safer.

This chapter offers examples of how to make your life easier by doing things in new ways. You can develop systems that work for you.

Storing or tossing

For people with declining vision, it is especially important to get started on downsizing and organizing before it becomes more difficult to see what you are dealing with. Another reason for doing the weeding now is that, if you don't do it yourself, someone else will end up doing it later. Is that what you'd want?

Before you get to work on organizing what you have, get rid of anything you don't need. Sort through your closets and drawers, and toss or give away things you do not use.

Weeding out clothing

If you have "vintage" or valuable clothing that is in good condition, you can take it to a consignment shop. Or, your children may want some of these items. In many communities, charitable organizations will pick up clothing (and, sometimes, household items and furniture that you no longer want). The point is to clear out your closets, bureau drawers, and shelves of things you no longer use. This leaves fewer things to search through when looking for something.

Keepsakes and photos

When going through your mementos, set aside things you think your children or other loved ones would like to have. It would be even better to have one of them help you with this task, because seeing precious things that have been stashed away can be an emotional experience. What may seem a difficult undertaking can be turned into a special time with a child when you share the history of an item that has sentimental meaning.

When organizing photos, you might want to go through them with family members and tell them a bit of family history or remember happy occasions together. Write the names of the people in the photo on the back and add a date for future identification. Have your favorite photos enlarged, or scan for permanent files you can send to children and friends.

Perhaps the most difficult task is to sort through letters and cards you have been keeping. It helps to be in the right mood—this is a sentimental task, and one that may be best done by you alone.

<hr>

MY STORY

Farewell to My "Dating" Dresses

My daughter learned a lot about me when I told her my history with each dress in an old closet in the basement. I hadn't looked at them in twenty years and dreaded seeing their condition after all that time in improper storage. Without the support of my daughter, I could not have gone through that closet. Actually, she was the one who took the dresses down from the clothes rod, one by one. I was not up to the task. I hated to think how my precious dresses might look. Each elicited a story, mostly about a special date with her father, occasions that remained vivid memories. She was enthralled to hear about the early days of her dad and me.

Remembering those happy times was an emotional and nostalgic experience, especially because my husband had died only a few weeks earlier. I was also sad to see that the dresses were now full of holes. My daughter convinced me that there was no point in hanging onto them. We should take care of matters then and there. I made my sad farewells. My daughter then directed me to go take a nap. After I got up, the dresses were gone. She had taken care of their disposal out of my view, for which I was thankful. I learned what, for me, was a hard lesson—that I don't need the actual object to keep its cherished memory. Realizing this has helped me in sorting through and discarding other items that were once important to me.

Everything in its place

As you proceed with weeding, start finding places for everything you want to keep. If there are groups of items that are difficult to see, find a new place to put them.

Finding things in drawers

Try to keep clothing you use frequently, such as underwear and socks, in an upper, easily reached drawer of a bureau where it is less difficult to see what's in the drawer and reach for what you want. It can become almost impossible to see items in a bottom drawer because lighting is poor near the floor, and bending over may be difficult. For me, even a flashlight does not help, but white shelf liner may offer enough contrast to identify items. If there is furniture in your bedroom with high drawers, but a partner with better vision is using them, try to make a trade of a couple of drawers or pieces of furniture.

Boxes are a help in organizing and finding things in drawers—and many other places. Be on the lookout for boxes that fit inside your drawers. Shoe boxes work well for small items—you can put particular colors of underwear or socks in them. If you find a particular kind of sock you like or an undergarment that fits just right, think about stocking up on that item so you have a supply and won't need to shop later and perhaps find that the product is no longer available.

Arranging clothes in closets

If you're like me and have a plain, old-fashioned closet with clothes rods, but no fancy organizers, these tricks are helpful, and they don't cost anything. Of course, the first step is to get rid of all those clothes you haven't worn recently. Then you can organize the remaining clothing. You may start with one method and later need a different way to identify colors.

Experiment to find what works best for you. Here are some ideas.

- Use white garments to separate the various colors of tops and shirts. The colors of my clothes are organized in my closet in this way: white, pink, white, black, white, blue, white, brown.

- A belt looped over the rod and then buckled is another good separator. It not only separates colors, the big loop makes the belt easy to find. I use an old white woven belt to separate my black and brown pants.

- When certain items go only with each other, hang them side by side.

- Leave the white paper on hangers from the dry cleaners to provide color contrast, making it easier to see what is on the hanger.

- Use colored plastic hangers or padded hangers in various designs. You can hang blue tops on blue hangers, brown on brown—or, for contrast, brown tops on beige hangers and beige tops on brown hangers.

- There is also the "safety pin method." This system can be used for all types of clothing, from shirts and pants to jackets and dresses. Use safety pins to identify colors by fastening a certain number of pins in the back labels or side tabs of each color of clothing. Because black is the most common color, leave black clothes free of safety pins—that can be their code. Here is an example of the system.

Black—no pin
Brown—one pin
Navy—two pins
Green—three pins

Shoes can be difficult to identify by color, especially if you have the same style in more than one color. I use a clothes pin to clip together my brown shoes to differentiate them from the identical black shoes. I no longer go out with unmatched shoes, which friends kindly wait to tell me about until I'm home. Another method is to keep a pair of shoes in its box.

Color-identifying devices

There are several models of devices that can announce over 150 different colors, such as Light Red and Vivid Red. They can be used to identify the color of clothing and for sorting laundry. But they are expensive and list many more colors than the basic ones most people need. If you want to try an electronic device, a free alternative is to download an app for your smart phone.

Organizing jewelry

If you have lots of earrings, pins, necklaces, or other jewelry, sort out the things you wear frequently. Try these ideas for organizing them.

Use an inexpensive plastic organizer, available at craft stores, and put different-colored earrings and other small jewelry pieces in the transparent compartments. For my earrings and small pins, my organizer has fourteen small compartments in two rows. Each row locks separately, and each compartment has a tight lid that won't open until the row is unlocked by pushing a little button on the side. Several pairs of earrings can fit into each compartment.

Another idea is to use small boxes. Place jewelry of the same color in each box, put a note on top with the name of the color, and secure with a rubber band. You may find a different system makes sense to you. Be a creative problem solver in finding systems that work to you—not just for jewelry but in all areas of your life.

Small items in small boxes

A great idea—that can be used in every room—is to use boxes to hold small, frequently used items such as dental floss, lip balm, night cream, comb, razor, and shaving lotion. Use a box that is large enough to hold the items in one layer so nothing is buried. This avoids the frustration in trying to find things inside the dark medicine cabinet, or scattered somewhere around the vanity.

Organizing medicine cabinets

Start organizing your medicine cabinet by disposing of items you no longer use and medications that have passed their expiration dates. Keep bottles of pills and other medicines and supplements that you take regularly, such as the AREDS formula for macular degeneration, in a special place where they'll be handy. Over-the-counter medicines that you take occasionally are handier if kept in your bathroom cabinet. Arrange like products such as lotions, hair and nail care products, and other personal care products together or on separate shelves, if available. Place each item in a special place so you will always be able to find it.

Filling prescriptions

Save time and trouble getting refills by asking your doctor to write each prescription for a three-month period, if paying for the larger quantity fits your budget. See if your pharmacy offers large print labels. I have asked my pharmacy to use easy opening caps, because I can't see where to line up the cap and the bottle on the regular caps.

Cutting pills in half

If you need to cut pills in half, an easy method is to use a scissors placed on the score line. Or use a pill cutter with a built-in magnifier, available at low vision stores. A plastic lid over the blade keeps the cut pieces from flying about. Still, this is a job you may prefer someone else to do. Some pharmacists will cut the pills for you.

Did I take my pills?

Solve the problem of remembering to take your medications at the correct times each day by using pill organizers. Organizers are available at drugstores and at low vision stores.

- If you take meds only in the morning and evening, it is handy to use two seven-compartment organizers, with slots for each day of the week. Get different-colored organizers for morning and evening.

- If you take meds three or four times a day, an organizer with four rows and twenty-eight compartments allows you to get all your meds for the week into one container.

- There are many different sizes, colors, and configurations of organizers—there's even one with an alarm system if needed.

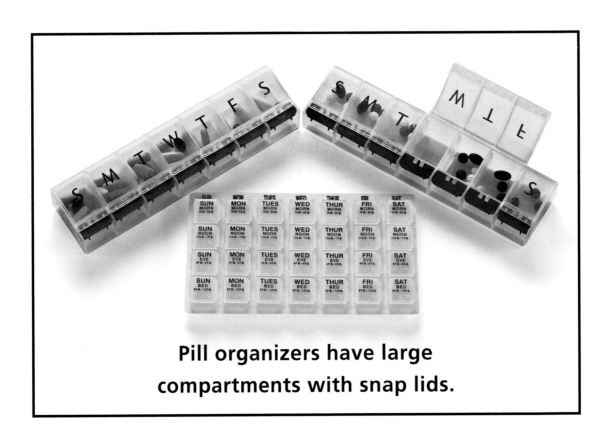

Pill organizers have large
compartments with snap lids.

- Store the bottles of pills that you take regularly in a plastic zip bag so they are handy when you are ready to fill your pill containers.

Avoid bouncing or dropping pills

It is easy to drop pills on the floor while transferring them from the bottles to the right compartments in the organizer. Stop the spill by sitting at a table and placing a terrycloth towel under the organizer so that, if you drop a pill, it does not bounce onto the floor. Begin with all the bottles still in the plastic bag. As you finish putting each bottle's pills in their compartments, close that bottle and place it on the table. When the plastic bag is empty, you'll know you have used all the bottles, and you won't have to wonder if you missed a medication. The weekly ritual of filling the pill containers can be a difficult and frustrating task, and at some point you may want to get help.

Kitchen organization

You can make things easier to find in your kitchen by organizing your cupboards, refrigerator, and freezer. Canned goods can be difficult to identify. It's not difficult to tell a can of soup from a can of tuna, but identifying the kind of soup that's in the can is another matter. Here are some tricks to try. Use various numbers of rubber bands on different kinds of soup, with no band for your favorite soup— let's say tomato, then one rubber band around chicken noodle soup, and two around vegetable beef. You can use the same system for canned vegetables. Index cards with the kind of soup in large dark letters can be wrapped around soup cans with rubber bands. Another technique is to place magnets with large letters on top of cans. If you don't have many varieties of canned goods, you can identify the cans by placing them in assigned locations on the shelf.

Refrigerator and freezer organizing

If you live with other people, designate one shelf in the refrigerator for any special food you may like or need for a special diet. Arrange items so that each one has a regular place. Use the same system in the freezer—everything in its place.

In your dish cupboard, put the most frequently used items on the lowest, most accessible shelf. For me, this means glasses and cups are on the bottom shelf. The next shelf has dinner and smaller plates of two sizes. The top shelf contains everyday bowls for cereal and soup, along with some heavy glass salad bowls that were a gift from a special friend. Reaching that top shelf is quite a stretch for me. It had been some time since I'd been able to see what is in the cupboards even in daylight.

—— MY STORY ——

A Broken Bowl

One dark evening I remembered I still needed to empty the dishwasher. I wanted to finish the job before my son came back to pick up his dog after he did some errands. The artificial lighting did not reach inside the cupboard; but that had not been a problem, because I knew the place for each item. I reached to the top shelf with one of the good salad bowls, but didn't realize the stack was tipping. The bowl crashed off the shelf, smashing into hundreds of small pieces that landed on the counter and, mostly, the floor.

I didn't want my son to know about my accident, so I started to pick up the pieces myself—a difficult task when I couldn't see them. I got out the broom and swept up some pieces, but I knew others had landed on the rug way over in front of the sink. It was too much for me to handle, so I knew I'd have to ask my son to take care of the rug—and to pick up the glass shards I was sure I'd missed on the counter and the floor.

I was frustrated and angry with myself. When my son finally arrived, he could tell by my stricken face that something was wrong. When I told him what had happened, instead of being annoyed, he just started the cleanup. He found large pieces of glass on the counter. I was incredulous that I hadn't seen them. My son expressed no hint of aggravation as he made sure he had picked up each piece of glass. This experience really brought home the fact that it is not just the person with vision loss who needs the gift of patience.

White shelf liner to the rescue

The broken bowl taught me that I needed to rearrange my dishes and glasses, but I still had problems because it was difficult to see into the cupboard. Then I discovered white, non-adhesive shelf liner that is non-skid on the bottom and easy to lift up. It is available at discount and home center stores. With help, I placed the liner on the top of the shelves—and also underneath on the bottoms and the sides of the cupboard. The white liner added the needed brightness and contrast to see what is inside. No more broken bowls!

Seeing what is in my silverware drawer had also been a problem until I had the idea of lining the dark wood sections with the white shelf liner.

Safe passage at home

Good balance is needed even when walking in your own home, where most accidents occur. See pages 57–63 for ideas on how to improve your balance. Identify hazards that could block your way or cause you to trip or fall in your own living space, and move furniture to clear any narrow passageways. If there is a vision loss resource center in your community, it may offer a home evaluation that will spot possible obstacles and hazards and help you find a safer way to arrange your furniture. Loose rugs pose a danger for tripping when they can't be seen, especially if you've developed a shuffling walk and may hit the rug with your toe, resulting in a fall. The safest policy is to remove area rugs.

Climbing stairs

Follow these guidelines when walking up or down stairs.

- Always use the handrail, but consider it a support only—not an indication that you are at the last step. Some handrails end before you get to the bottom.

- Know the number of steps in the stairs you use every day, and count as you go up and down, so you know where you are.

- If you have a weak leg, lead with the "bad" leg when going down and the "good" leg when going up. Bring your second leg to the same step once the first is firmly in place. For the next step, lead with the same leg you used before—do not alternate legs. Remember the rule that the "bad" leg leads going down the stairs, and the "good" leg leads going up.

To mark the bottom and top step, apply yellow and black striped hazard tape to mark the first and last steps of your stairs, corners, cabinet edges, etc. The tape comes in a roll and is adhesive on one side. It adheres to both wood and carpeted steps and is available at home center stores. My roll is 2" by 18 yards. I also tried reflective safety tape, but for me it was not as visible as the much cheaper non-reflective hazard tape. Good lighting is required to see the tape.

For even greater visibility, I ran patio string lights, also available at home center stores, down both sides of my staircase and continuing to my light switch. My set, called "48 ft incandescent Rope Light Kit," has lights incased one inch apart in heavy-duty PVC. This single change has given me a great sense of safety living alone in my own home.

Using the telephone

If you have a landline phone, avoid the dangers of rushing to answer the phone by placing phones in convenient locations. Ideally, have a phone in every room. This is possible with a cordless system that comes with multiple handsets, which only require one of the phones in a set to be connected to a phone jack.

Sometimes the only way to have a phone in a handy place is to run a phone line along the floor. If this absolutely cannot be avoided, cover the line with heavy shipping tape or duct tape so you do not trip on the loose cord.

A cell phone is another possibility, especially if you can keep it with you at all times—and remember to keep it charged. Many cell phones have features that allow you to place calls with a voice command, an extremely helpful feature. See Chapter 13 for a description of special low vision accessibility options.

9

Find Hard-to-Spot Things

DO THINGS VANISH after you have set them down somewhere? Do you have problems finding things because you can't see them on a counter or table? Is it difficult to get your house key into the keyhole, especially at night when it's dark? Learn how to use contrast and your sense of touch to solve these problems.

Tactile bumps and marks

To identify objects, small, raised, plastic "bumps" are among the most useful things in my life. Available at low vision stores, these bumps adhere to most surfaces, and they make it possible to find all sorts of things by touch.

Two types of bumps are available. The first are round or square raised bumps that are flat on the bottom and coated with a strong adhesive. They come in a variety of sizes, colors, and materials. In addition, there are flat stick-ons made of felt, velour, and cork. They come in darker colors than the plastic bumps and provide different textures to the touch.

By using a variety of sizes, colors, and textures, you can distinguish things, such as different buttons on a remote control or special keys on a computer keyboard. For example, I've marked the "delete" key of my computer keyboard with a round clear bump, and the "Enter" key is marked with a flat brown stick-on. The center "F" and "J" keys have bumps so I can correctly place my fingers on the keyboard, which vastly improves my typing accuracy. The cost of the bumps is minimal. They come in packs of ten to forty, depending on the size and material. The other type of bump is a raised dot made with a special paint pen on surfaces where permanent dots are needed or where adhesive dots do not stick. These raised dots are useful on such items as metal measuring cups and stove dials. See page 88–89 for a photo and description of how to apply them.

Over the years, I've added the adhesive-backed plastic bumps to more and more items. In my kitchen, I use them on the dishwasher's power button and on the microwave oven "one minute" and power level buttons. On the TV remote control, I have bumps on the power, volume, and "channel up" buttons. Meanwhile, I've used the paint pens to create high marks on my VCR remote control and to draw raised lines on my coffee carafe at the levels I frequently use.

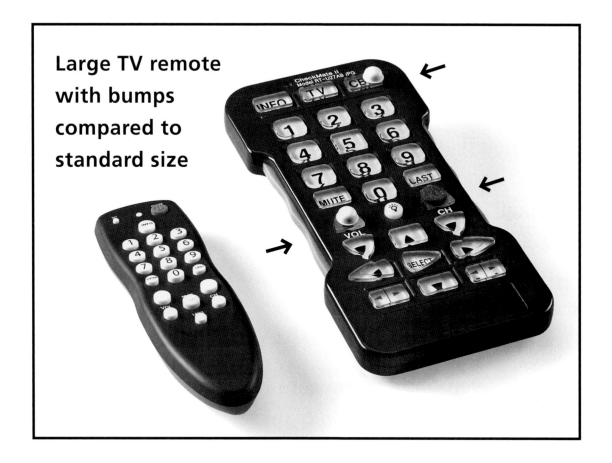

Large TV remote with bumps compared to standard size

Bumps and high marks can be placed on any number of items—telephone buttons, computer power switches, telephones, dishwashers, clothes washer dials, remote controls, and other items you want to recognize by touch. Analyze your own needs; then get busy marking items you want to be able to find more easily.

Purse, briefcase, and backpack

Trying to find something in a purse, briefcase, or backpack can be like looking into a deep, black hole. Avoid a carryall that is one big pocket, and instead get one that has two or three main compartments and some little pockets in at least one of the compartments. Then figure out what goes in each section, and stick to your plan. My purse has multiple pockets that I use for my cell phone, my wallet, and for small items such as pens, cards, and keys. My flashlight is large and easy to feel, so it goes in the bottom of a large pocket.

Bold pens make it easy

Reading even one's own writing becomes more and more difficult as sight diminishes. At first it is easy to read handwriting in pencil, but eventually you can make out only writing done in ink. Then even writing done in black ink can be tough to read. Felt-tip pens provide a darker line and are readily available in many types of stores. If you require an even darker, bolder line, the answer is a Sanford 20/20® pen. The pen is available at low vision stores. The ink just flows out of these pens without bleeding to the other side, and the writing is dark and easy to read.

To help spot the pen in a jar or box with other pens, or pens on a desk or countertop, I wrap a heavy rubber band around the top of the pen. I often find my pen by feel rather than sight—the rubber band works both ways. If it is difficult to read because your lines are not straight, use paper with wide lines 1" apart. I print these from my computer on a form I made.

Contrast makes items visible

- Put white doilies on the arms and backs of dark-colored chairs.
- Put contrasting throw pillows on the sofa.
- Cover coffee tables and side tables with bright fabric or something white—something that contrasts with the flooring color.

- Place a bright tablecloth or centerpiece on the dining room or kitchen table.

- Use yellow/black striped warning tape to mark corners, cabinet edges, etc., as well as the top and bottom of your stairs.

- Use light switch faceplates in colors that contrast with the colors of the walls.

- Put contrasting-colored knobs on cupboard doors and dresser drawers.

- Have a readily available light at the entrance to each room. If there is no light switch by the door, consider adding a lamp that you can turn on by clapping your hands.

- Put rubber bands around various objects to find by sight or touch.

- Place a dark 12" × 12" hardboard on a light kitchen countertop for any small item that is hard to spot. I can place light-colored notepaper on this surface as well to avoid mistakenly writing on my light-colored countertop.

- Try white bumps on a black stapler or TV control buttons.

- Try orange bumps on oven, washer, and dryer dials.

Checks with bold, raised lines

When it took me an hour one evening to write only three checks and then try to enter them in the check register, I decided it was time to get large print checks. Mine are about 8" across and 3¼" high. They have bold black raised lines, and the background is yellow to help reduce glare and provide contrast. They were available at my bank, and I was not charged for them.

Another option is to have someone else fill out regular checks, and then you sign them. If you have difficulty getting your signature to fit on the line, you can arrange with your bank to abbreviate your signature to just your first initial and last name. Another option is a check-writing guide, which is a template that is placed over a blank check. You write in the cutout slots that fit over the lines on the check. The guides are available at low vision stores.

You can avoid writing and signing checks entirely by doing what my mother and I did when she no longer could see well enough to write checks. She had me added to her checking account, and I handled all her bill paying from that point on. Now I'm following that tradition by adding my son to my checking account.

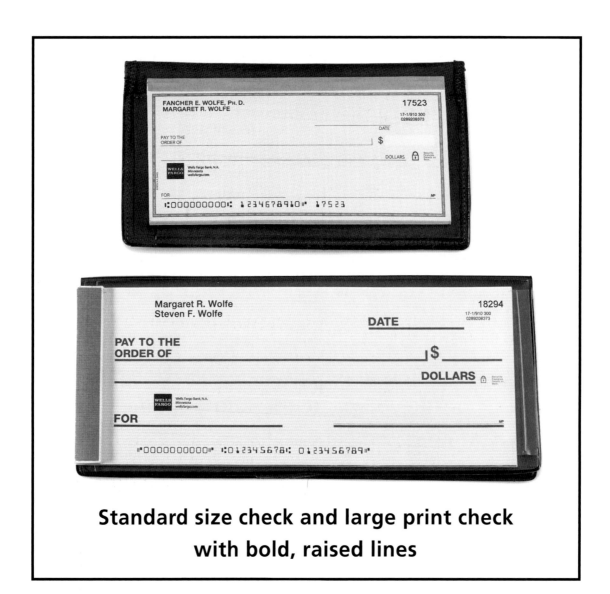

Standard size check and large print check
with bold, raised lines

Balancing your checkbook

Fitting dollar amounts in the columns on the regular
check registers provided by the bank is even more
difficult than writing the check. You can make your
own register by using a notebook with lined paper
and drawing columns for check number, date, payee,

check amount, deposit amount, and balance. You can also custom design a form on your computer and even track the balance on the document.

If you use large print checks from the bank, the check register provided is the same large size with wide spaces for entering the check data. Mine includes monthly calendars. Another solution is to buy a large print check register from a low vision store. The spaces are big enough to write in using a bold pen. Big-number and talking calculators are available to help you balance your check register.

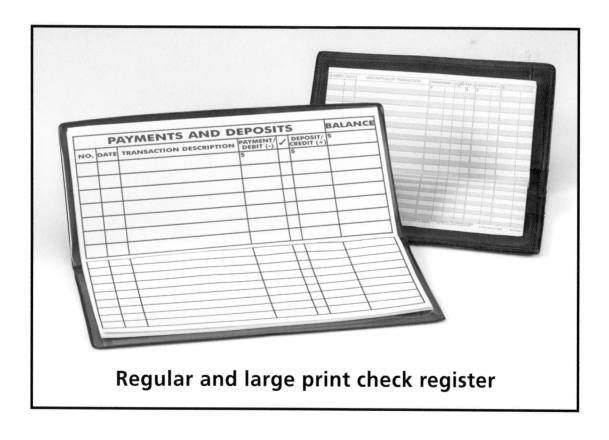

Regular and large print check register

Online banking for convenience

If you use a computer, you can manage your day-to-day finances from home. View a history of your transactions, transfer money between accounts, order checks. And, to avoid having to write checks, use automatic bill pay for recurring monthly bills, such as gas, electric, telephone, and mortgage. You may choose the date to have them paid to be a few days after your other regular deposits—such as a paycheck, pension, or Social Security—are deposited in your account. You can still receive printed statements (marked DO NOT PAY) from the various companies for these bills in the mail or as email attachments.

Debit and credit cards

You can cut down on the number of checks you need to write by using either a bank debit card (sometimes called a check card) or a traditional credit card. With each type of card you receive a monthly statement that itemizes the date and place of each purchase. This listing is handy for record keeping.

When using a debit card, the amount of your purchase is immediately deducted from your bank account. This offers convenience in that you do not have to write a check each month to cover your purchases as you do with a credit card. However, you will be charged an overdraft fee for purchases made when you do not have sufficient funds in your account. Overdraft charges are an unnecessary expense and add up quickly, so keep a record of the amount of each purchase in a register, and don't use the card if you do not have enough money in the account to cover your purchase. Insufficient bank funds may also result in a purchase being denied—this is not only embarrassing, but also an annoyance if you have to leave the store without the items you wanted to buy.

Before using a debit card, make sure you understand all the conditions of use. Have someone read you the terms or check with the issuer of the card if you have questions about the terms. Unlike issuers of credit cards, most banks do not protect you if your debit card is stolen and someone uses it to make purchases or get cash from an ATM machine. All the funds in your bank account could be wiped out, so guard your card carefully.

With a traditional credit card, you are sent a statement each month. If you do not pay the balance in full, you are charged an interest fee. To avoid additional debt from high interest rates, consider what you are able to afford and, if possible, do not charge more than you can pay off each month. If you use the credit card for all your purchases, you need to write only one check each month.

Plugging cords into receptacles

To avoid having to bend over or even crawl around the floor, trying to find receptacles, use power surge strips with cords that are long enough to allow you to place the strips in convenient places closer to eye level, such as on a side table.

Finding keyholes and inserting keys

This is such a foolproof method that it works even when it's dark and you don't know where the lock is on the door.

■ Find the key you want on the key ring. Hold it upright in your dominant hand. If there are ridges on only one side of the key, the flat part of the key is the bottom. If the key has ridges on both sides, it may be a bit tricky to figure out which way the key should be turned to go into the lock. You can add a dot on the top side with a paint pen.

- Find the lock by feel with your hand.

- With your fingertips, find the keyhole and place your thumbnail next to it.

- Place the key next to your thumbnail.

- Use your thumbnail to guide the key into the lock.

- Turn the key and the doorknob, and open the door.

Travel and Transportation

GETTING AROUND TOWN includes many modes: automobiles, walking, bicycling, public transportation by bus and rail, and private transportation in taxicabs. We may be able to drive our own cars; but if we have had to stop driving, we may receive rides from friends and relatives and perhaps use some other methods. Travel to other cities and countries can involve bus, train, boat, and airplane. There are many accommodations for traveling by these transportation modes. Safety must come first, no matter how we travel.

Driving our own cars is usually our first choice, but driving safely involves many factors and good vision is only one of them. Strength and agility are also needed because driving involves the use of most of the muscle groups in the body, as explained on page 63–64. Although loss of the ability to drive safely is one of the most difficult things to face, it can help to remember that even people with excellent vision may be forced to stop driving if they lack the health or motor skills required to safely operate an automobile.

Should I still be driving?

Safety—for you, your passengers, those in other vehicles, bikers, and pedestrians—must be the prime consideration when you decide whether or not it is all right for you to drive. Even if you still have a valid driver's license, you may decide that it is time to stop driving. Be honest with yourself, and you will be the best judge of if, when, and where you should be driving. Ask yourself these questions:

- Do I feel unsafe when I'm driving, even on familiar routes?

- Do vehicles or people seem to appear suddenly out of nowhere?

- Do I have physical issues, such as slow reaction time or inability to turn my head or my upper body, that hinder my ability to check for other vehicles?

- Are other people reluctant to get in the car with me when I'm the driver?

- Have family members or friends suggested that it's time I stop driving?

- Do I become panicky or lose confidence when I find myself in congested or fast-moving traffic?

If your answer to any of these questions is yes, it is time for you to consider whether you should limit or stop driving. To help you decide, occupational therapists and some rehabilitation centers offer professional assessments. Take charge of how to make the decision.

I'm driving for now

If you are still driving, consider adopting self-imposed restrictions such as not driving at night or when it is raining or snowing, staying within a comfortable speed limit, traveling only on local roads with which you are familiar, and canceling trips if the weather is threatening. Giving up driving can be a gradual process with such restrictions.

The driver's license vision test

When the time to renew your driver's license approaches, you may find it helpful to prepare for the vision test by following these tips. Because states vary in their minimum vision requirements for passing the test, cutoff points are not listed here.

- Plan to take the test a few weeks ahead of your birthday—don't wait until the last minute, when you may be more anxious about passing because of the deadline.

- Take the test on a day when both you and your eyes are feeling especially good—a day when you feel confident.

- Have someone drive you to the test so you don't become nervous just getting to the licensing bureau.

- Ask that your driver come in with you, as you might need help in filling out the renewal application form. When I recently applied, my son had to fill out the form because it was so dark at the writing table that I could not read the questions or write the answers.

A restricted license?

If you don't pass the test, you may be eligible for a restricted license if it is offered in your state. Besides wearing eyeglasses, restrictions can include no nighttime driving, no freeway driving, no driving beyond limited areas or routes, and no driving above a certain speed. Some states require a recommendation on restrictions from an eye doctor; others may determine restrictions at the licensing bureau.

Driver safety class

These classes are offered by many different organizations at a reasonable price. They are called by various names, including "Senior Driver Improvement Classes" (AAA) and "Driver Safety Program" (AARP), which offers an online course as well as classroom locations, such as community centers, senior centers, and churches. At least for the first time, attend a class in person. The give and take of class discussions alone is worth making the trip to the classroom.

The basic course is an eight-hour session that is usually offered in two four-hour segments, although sometimes an all-day course is offered on weekends. In most states, insurance rates are discounted for those who have taken such courses. Refresher courses, which generally consist of one four-hour session, can be taken as often as you wish, but to retain insurance discounts, the refresher course is generally required every three years.

In the class, you can expect to learn about current rules of the road, how to operate your vehicle more safely, and how to make some adjustments to common age-related changes in vision, hearing, and reaction time. Here is a list of some specific topics that may be covered.

- Maintaining the proper distance from other moving vehicles.

- Changing lanes and making turns at intersections in the safest ways.

- Knowing the effects of medications on driving ability.

- Minimizing the effects of dangerous blind spots.

- Eliminating driver distractions such as eating, smoking, and cell phone use.

- Proper use of seat belts, air bags, and antilock brakes.

- Continuing to monitor your own and others' driving skills and capabilities.

Prepare yourself and your car

Before you start off on your drive, prepare for the trip, even if it's a short trip to a familiar place. Use the checklist below to ensure that you are prepared before you get behind the wheel.

- Make sure you have the proper glasses for driving. If you have separate reading and distance glasses, get an extra pair of distance glasses to keep permanently in the car, and store them in a dedicated location.

- Keep a pair of sunglasses in a dedicated location in the car.

- Practice this trick for times when the sun is periodically blocked by clouds or when the sun is not bright at the start of a trip and wearing sunglasses would make the road look too dark. Keep your sunglasses handy by putting them above your regular glasses or on top of your head, and just slide them down when you're confronted with glare. Push them back up when the sunlight has diminished.

- Assess the weather and check weather forecasts. If rain or snow is falling or predicted, consider postponing the trip. You do not want to be stranded and unable to drive back home. If it is a sunny day and you are sensitive to glare even when wearing sunglasses, consider postponing your trip or finding another means of transportation.

- Put raised bumps on dashboard buttons, such as those for the heater and defroster, so you can quickly locate them by feel. Practice reaching for the bumps before you drive to see if you are able to find them quickly.

- Check your seat position and mirrors, and make adjustments if necessary.

- Show fuel levels by putting a white dot at the half-full or quarter-full level.

Driving the car—safety pointers

- Stay alert at all times.
- Do what you need to do to feel safe.

- Concentrate on the cars ahead, but glance periodically at the side and rear mirrors.

- Know your weak spots, such as slow reaction time or the need for lots of light, and drive accordingly.

- Stay fit and flexible—all parts of the body are involved in driving.

- Plan to be home before dark. Check the time of sunset, estimate how long you will be gone, add a half hour for delays, and then work backward to figure out when you must drive home in order to get there before dusk.

"Later" has arrived: giving up the keys

Giving up driving is actually a gradual process. Long before you make the decision not to drive at all, you will probably have placed you own restrictions on your driving: no driving at night, no driving on freeways, then only short trips in your neighborhood. You may have had to cancel a trip or find a ride when the weather or other factors prevented you from driving. But the "final" day is typically long dreaded. You be the one to make the reasonable decision about when that day has arrived. Being responsible for yourself is a form of independence and preserves your dignity. It also prevents a "taking away the keys" scene with your children or friends, or law enforcement officials.

Ideas that make it easier

- Add up the cost of gasoline, car repairs, and automobile insurance for the previous year. That is the amount that you saved. Now you can spend that amount on taxicabs or public transportation each year, with no additional expense to your overall budget.

- Make these savings a special fund. Use a "taxi jar" for ready cash.

- If you sell your car, realize that those proceeds are a one-time windfall. Rather than adding the amount to the taxi jar, consider putting it in a "fun fund" for trips for yourself—not for doctor's appointments or other trips made out of necessity.

- When you happen to get a ride with a taxi driver you like, ask for his or her card, and call directly when you need a ride. You may find an important new friend in your life.

- Look for a private driver—sometimes a person right in your neighborhood would welcome the opportunity to take you on errands or trips—and may charge much less than a commercial cab with set rates.

- Ask for rides from relatives and friends, and think of favors to do in return, such as paying for parking, buying a few gallons of gas or a fun gift, or treating them to dinner at a nice restaurant.

Door-to-door transit services

In many communities there are low cost transportation services that are available as mandated by the Americans with Disabilities Act of 1990. Besides the low cost, another advantage is that the driver comes to your door and assists you in getting into and out of the car or van. There may be other passengers. There is usually an application process to become eligible for these services. See page 181.

Another possibility is to check with Medicaid, if you are in the program, to see if costs of transportation services to get you to medical appointments are covered. If your community has a good public transit system, you have yet another alternative for transportation.

Now relax and enjoy your trips as a passenger. Relish the peace of mind that both you and your loved ones have knowing that you are safe when on the road.

Use a white cane?

If you are accustomed to walking to nearby locations, make sure you are able to see oncoming cars and traffic lights. If your vision loss has declined to the point where you do not feel safe when you walk, consider getting instruction on the use of a white cane in orientation and mobility training. It is a good signal to drivers that you may need extra time to cross the street. See page 180 for more information.

————— **MY STORY** —————

Taxi Al, Clark, and Barry

Two weeks after passing the vision test for my seventy-seventh birthday driver's license renewal, I noticed a loss of vision in my right eye. I had already become more careful about where to drive; but after learning there was bleeding in my eye and receiving an injection as treatment, I had to reassess my ability to drive at all. A couple of weeks earlier, I had called a taxicab company when I needed a ride to a doctor's appointment that would have required me to drive on an unfamiliar freeway. I immediately liked the driver who answered the call, so I asked if he could pick me up after the appointment and if I could arrange rides with him ahead of time. He handed me a card that read, "TAXI-AL at your service." I discovered that he lived close by me and was able to schedule trips far in advance if I called him directly.

Two days later, Taxi Al took me to my volunteer job. I started to schedule trips with him weeks in advance. We became good friends, and it was a comfort to have him waiting for me after a difficult medical procedure. He had an arrangement with two other drivers, and if he couldn't make a trip, he arranged for Clark or Barry to pick me up. When Taxi Al took a job out of town, he turned me over to my new steady driver, "Taxi Clark." He will take me anywhere at any time—to the airport at 5:00 a.m. and to the veterinarian with me and three dogs, the best behaved sitting up in front with him. Clark and Barry have a backup arrangement, so if Clark can't make a trip, he lets me know that Barry will do the trip. These men are good friends who are indispensable to me.

Other drivers in my life

Then there is my longstanding arrangement with my friend Arlys. We have held season orchestra tickets since 1990, and she became the driver many years ago when I could no longer drive at night. I'm not far out of her way, but it is still a detour. To show my appreciation, I pay for the parking and sometimes treat her to dinner. She is happy with the arrangement, and our bonus is that all those hours spent together in the car have firmly cemented our friendship.

Another regular driver came from an unexpected source. Reiko, my ballet teacher, knew I'd missed a class because of threatening rain. (I do not take the chance of being stranded because of a rainstorm.) She asked Amy, who lives near me, to start taking me to and from a summer class, which was held some distance from my home. Because Reiko made this arrangement without consulting me, I was upset and not the least bit gracious. In fact, I called her a mother hen (now we laugh about that). Amy insisted it would be her pleasure to drive me to class and back, but I found that hard to believe. Although it was difficult to admit to myself that I should no longer make that drive, it was even harder to accept unsolicited help. This was a new role for me, and one I am still adjusting to. It has helped that Amy and I enjoy our time together and that we have become fast friends during our trips. In summer months her teen daughters join us, and it's been a delight to have these young friends and to hear all about their lives.

My son is also an important driver. He comes to work in our home office every weekday and, although we have agreed that I will not ask him to use his work time to drive me long distances, he does run short errands for me and does the grocery shopping. I do not feel reluctant to ask

Out-of-town travel

There are two parts to travel away from home— getting there and upon arrival settling into unfamiliar surroundings. Assert your independence by being a self-advocate. Always feel free to ask for help—from taxi and bus drivers, hotel clerks, airline personnel, or ship crews.

Airplane tips

- When you are buying the ticket, get a seat near the front, request any special help options you will need such as a wheelchair to take you to your gate so you won't have to find your way around the airport.

- Pre-ship your suitcase by a ground service. Depending on its weight and destination, it may not cost much more than the airline cost of checking your bag, and it will be waiting for you at your final destination. Avoid the hassle at the airport of checking or carrying your bag, or waiting for your suitcase at the baggage carousel.

- At the airport, for extra help, ask for customer service personnel. If you feel that you have been treated unfairly, then ask for a Complaints Resolution official (CRO). CROs have been trained in disability options.

- Use a cell phone to take a photo of gate listings and then enlarge on the phone.

- Ask for an escort to take you through security and to your gate, and then alert them that at your destination that you will need an escort to go to baggage, a new gate, or customs.

- Preboard.

- Notify flight attendant of your visual impairment, in case of an emergency.

Hotel tips

- Ask for a room on the first floor so you don't have to locate floor buttons on the elevator.

- If there are no rooms on first floor, ask for a room next to the elevator so you don't have to count a lot of room doors.

- Put a raised dot by your floor button in the elevator, and remove it when you leave.

- At check in, ask hotel staff to take you to your room to—

    put a raised white dot near the key slot.
    turn on lights and show locations of switches.
    show locations of room phone and TV control (and how it works).
    set up the coffeemaker.

- If the hotel has a concierge, make acquaintance and tip if you used services.

Hot Coffee—and No Spills

When settling into my hotel room while attending a retreat at a nearby center, I realized I was not able to read the directions on the in-room coffeemaker. How was I to have my three cups of morning coffee, I wondered in a panic. Then, when I was unpacking, my eyes fell on something I'd thrown into my suitcase at the last minute—with no specific purpose in mind. It was a small bag from an eyeglass store that opened to a flat bottom about 6" across. The bag had a rope handle.

In the morning I had an inspiration—I grabbed the bag and went down to the lobby where coffee was available from a large urn. I couldn't see its handle, but a kind person, who I later saw at the retreat, offered to fill a cup when I explained I couldn't see well. Then he asked if I wanted a lid. Yes, what a wonderful idea! Then I realized two more cups would fit in the bag, and my helper obliged. When I got to the door of my room, I hooked the handle of the bag over my arm. With two free hands, I felt for the bump I'd put near the key slot with one hand and inserted the key with the other. I entered the room and saw there were no spills. Coffee was never so appreciated as I sipped it in my room.

From now on, there will always be a coffee-carrying bag in my suitcase!

Tours for easy travel

If you want to go on a sightseeing trip, consider joining a tour. Everything will be taken care of, from ordering your airplane tickets to making all baggage transfers to making hotel reservations. Experienced tour guides will offer commentary as you ride along in your bus. You will meet people and make new friends.

There are special tours for people with low vision. See a list by doing an Internet search on "low vision tours."

11

Accept Help

OPEN YOUR HEART AND YOUR MIND to the prospect of reaping great rewards by accepting help. This can be a difficult adjustment to make. Needing others can make you feel powerless, but you maintain independence by being the one who chooses if and when to seek or accept that help. Your friends and family can learn the best ways to help you if you are open to explaining your needs. Open communication is key. Let them know if it may be difficult for you to ask for help.

Be assertive in finding what type of outside assistance is available in your area. You may start with special recreation events and transportation services. Professional help is available that offers training for maintaining as much independence as possible. The entire next chapter is devoted to this specialty: vision rehabilitation.

Explain your needs

Share your feelings with family and friends. Let them know that there will be times when you need to call on them for help, but that you are in charge of your own life and are exploring the resources available to people with vision loss. Your vision loss affects not only you, but your family and friends, too. Realize that they must also develop a spirit of acceptance and patience. They may need to help you with various tasks, but let that help be in ways that are appropriate and useful for you. If you are not the instigator of the idea of such help, you may feel a loss of control. Maintain independence by deciding what help you want to accept and when you want to actively seek help in a particular area of your life. This will help you maintain the satisfaction that comes with being actively in control of your life.

Handling various "help" situations

Sometimes family and friends do not know how to give you the help you may—or may not—need. It is up to you to let them know what is right for you. Here are examples of ways to handle situations with certain types of people.

- Overly protective people may offer unsolicited help that you do not need or want. You can be politely assertive and say, "It's important that I stay as independent as possible, so please allow me do whatever I can. I'll ask for assistance when I need it, so don't feel you always need to offer help."

- Those who are oblivious to your situation often ignore the fact that you need assistance in some area—the opposite of being too solicitous. Again it is up to you to let them know what you need. You can say, "I appreciate your thinking I can do everything myself, but I would like your help with (you name it)."

- People attuned to your needs and desires are the ideal helpers, so ask for and accept their help with thanks.

- Be aware of being stubborn and rejecting help that you could actually use but refuse because you'd then have to admit that you need it. This has much less to do with other people than it does with you. Ask yourself, "Am I letting pride or denial or stubbornness get in the way of acting in my own best interests?" If the answer is yes, try not to become huffy, as I did (and came to regret) when I didn't want to accept a ride, as described on pages 152–154.

Accepting too much help

If someone in your life is a very helpful type, it is easy to fall into the trap of accepting or asking for help that you do not really need. Doing so will ultimately reduce your independence. In my own case, I strive to be more aware so I don't automatically use help from my son for things that I don't actually need. He comes to work every weekday in the home office of our family publishing business. He is patient and kind; and, if I'm looking for something I've set down somewhere, I can get frustrated and ask him to find it rather than keep searching for it myself.

Sometimes when I find myself too easily accepting or relying on assistance with some task I could safely accomplish on my own, I remember a gentleman who attended the low vision skills class I took. He had very little vision and his wife drove him to class, but she did not hang around during the class to assist him—

instead, she went upstairs, did crossword puzzles, and came back in time to join in the lunch we prepared in class. She reminded him that he was in the class to learn to do things for himself. She was reinforcing his need for independence, and she let him know that she was not going to help him when he could do something for himself. This example serves as a good reminder to be conscious of the type of help we are using and to make sure it is at an appropriate level.

Be proactive—voice your needs

These examples may seem difficult to follow at first, but with practice you will feel more and more comfortable advocating for yourself. Develop your can-do, independent attitude that will fuel your self-confidence and hopeful outlook.

- Be open about telling people how you are feeling so they don't have to try to guess whether or not something is wrong.

- If you are having a bad eye day (or, as one woman puts it, "My eyes are crabby today"), you may need to ask for special attention or help in deciding whether or not you want to participate in a planned activity.

- Feel free to suggest things you would really like from others, such as offers to take you shopping or to a doctor appointment, or fun things like going out to lunch, or the opportunity to share gift ideas that you have found in low vision catalogs.

Be direct and polite when asking for help

It is vital to clearly state exactly what help you are requesting. I was horrified to learn that, for years, the way I asked my son for help was actually irritating—without my realizing it.

———— MY SON'S STORY ————

Christmastime Outburst

The whole family was in town; and my mother had been in a tizzy for days, trying to get her cards in the mail before Christmas. I was already feeling stressed two days before Christmas, trying to find time to finish my holiday shopping.

Mom and I were looking at recipes, trying to decide on a menu for dinner. Whenever she came across an ingredient that we didn't have on hand, she would point it out in a *"Woe is me, I can't drive to the store"* voice.

After a few minutes of this, I exploded, telling her that she should just ask me outright if she wants help. When I feel that I am being manipulated into making an offer to do something, I feel put upon and get defensive. If I am just asked directly to do something, even it is a chore, I would be glad to help.

Since Mom and I altered our way of communicating in situations like this, I have felt more willing to help out, and I stay in a good mood while doing it.

—— MY STORY ——

"Poor Peggy"

I was stunned by my son's words! I had believed for years that I must first try to do something myself before I am justified in asking for help. Only then would I call out, in a voice that I now learned came across as whiny and "Poor Peggy," saying, "I've been trying to find the postage stamps in this drawer for ten minutes; and I'm very annoyed, but have to give up. I just can't see into the drawer anymore. Can you interrupt what you're doing and come here right away and find the stamps for me?"

Now I've learned to say, "Steve, I need a stamp. Can you please come and find one for me?" I guard against becoming demanding, even when feeling frustrated. I try to always be polite and appreciative.

Thanks to Steve's words, I have a happier, more open relationship with my son—and this is precious to me.

———————

Talk about your vision loss?

Sometimes when you are out and about, you may run into situations in which it makes sense to mention that you have a vision loss. Remember that, in all cases, it is up to you to decide whether or not you want to say anything. Here are some scenarios and ideas for how you could handle them.

- At a store, you may need help with reading a price tag, or with signing for a charge at the checkout station when you can't see where to write your signature. Practice a standard line that you can say with confidence, such as, "Please show me where to sign, as I don't see well (or have vision loss, or have poor vision," or my short phrase, "I have bad eyes."

- At social gatherings and other situations, if you are open about your vision, you may have some interesting conversations when the person you are talking with tells you all about a relative or friend with vision loss. I've made some wonderful new connections this way.

- If people become overly inquisitive, remember that you are under no obligation to talk about your vision. You can say, "I prefer not to discuss this," or, "I find it rather boring to discuss my vision loss."

Develop a spirit of gratitude

As we continue to make adjustments in our lives to accommodate vision loss we can experience many feelings, but gratitude may not readily come to mind, yet it is an important gift to both you and others. Try to remember to thank the helpers in your life. Let them know you appreciate what they do for you. Recognize that your situation makes life difficult for them, too.

Sometimes I think I present a triple whammy to those around me. I have vision loss and need help in many areas. I have a hearing loss—and I don't always wear my hearing aids, so I'm often saying, "What? Can you say that again more clearly?" I also have celiac disease and can't eat a normal diet—no wheat, oats, barley, or rye. My family and friends have immense kindness and patience in the ways they must adapt their lives to fit my needs, yet how often do I remember to let them know how grateful I am for their help?

Use local resources

Besides your immediate circle of family and friends, there are local resources in many cities that can offer help and a variety of services in the areas of recreation, transportation, and healthcare. In addition to the special adaptive recreational opportunities described below, assistive services are offered by a wide array of senior centers and community centers. Some cities have vision loss agencies that offer a variety of social and recreational activities, in addition to training. Such organizations are described in the next chapter, Vision Rehabilitation.

Adaptive recreational opportunities

Audio descriptions of the visual elements of live theater, selected television shows, and some movies are available to enhance your understanding and enjoyment of these types of entertainment.

- Television. Descriptions by a narrator of visual elements such as actions, settings, scene changes, and body language are provided during natural breaks in the program's dialog. Check with your local stations or cable companies to see what is available. Also, when buying a new television set, be sure that it can accept audio description.

- Audio-described performance. Theater productions of plays that run for long periods of time (as opposed to those that open and close quickly or that come into town for a day or two) often have performances that include audio descriptions. You wear a headset to hear the narration, which takes place when nothing is being spoken on stage. Ticket prices are often subsidized for you and a companion. Call your local theater companies to find out if they have these performances.

- Audio-described movies and videos. Visit the following websites to locate movie theaters that show audio-described films by country, state, and city. Call local movie theaters to ask if they show audio-described movies.

- A list of audio-described movies with ratings on the ease or difficulty of following the story is offered by the website Blindspots: Movie Reviews for Visually Impaired People (www.vashti.net/Blind/table.htm)

Talking books and magazines

You can borrow recorded books, magazines, and playback equipment from a regional library that is in the network of the Talking Book program of the National Library Service for the Blind and Physically Handicapped (NLS). See more on pages 49–52.

Transportation services

Information on transportation services for the disabled is described on page 149. To find transportation services in your area, contact your local Area Agency on Aging by calling 1-800-677-1116.

A Weekend Asking Strangers for Help

With great trepidation, I accepted an invitation to a retreat on friendship, even though I had no way to get to the location 250 miles away that had no bus or plane service. I would be staying at a strange hotel in a room by myself, and wouldn't know a single soul among the forty registrants. The sessions were to be held in a retreat center in a large building with a spread-out design and multiple levels. All this was scary. I'd be off on my own, not knowing a single person, yet need to ask strangers for all sorts of help. Could I get up my courage to be so outgoing and assertive? I could hardly believe it when I registered for the retreat. It would have been a daunting venture for me even if I had perfect vision.

The first step was finding a way to get there. I called the director of the retreat, Mary, and she told me she would contact Ellen, who was driving from my city. She agreed to take me, but was not coming directly back home. Mary offered to drive me home herself. I protested that I couldn't possibly accept such a generous offer, but agreed when she said she'd combine the trip with a visit to her sister who lived near me. Now there was no turning back.

On the six-hour drive to the retreat with Ellen, we became great friends. When we stopped at the hotel, we met another woman attending the retreat and chatted briefly. Ellen was not staying in the hotel, but she helped me get settled in my room. I used many tips for staying alone in a hotel room, described in Chapter 10, Travel and Transportation.

When we attended the first session at the retreat that evening, Ellen sat in the back. I had to leave her to sit in the front row so I could better see the two presenters. I was the second person called upon to stand and tell something about myself, but I didn't mention my vision loss. After the session, there was a social hour. I knew the time was drawing near when I would have to find a ride back to the hotel. I felt uncomfortable having to ask a stranger for such help, but I thought of the woman I'd met in the hotel lobby. I remembered only that she was tall and thin—one of the ways I identify people because I can't recognize faces.

Again I had to ask for help—in order to ask for more help. Ellen found me standing perplexed. I told her my idea but said I couldn't find the woman I wanted to ask. Ellen spotted her right away. She read her name tag and told me her name was Donna. I felt intimidated, but knew I had to ask for her help because I had to get back to the hotel. I explained my vision loss, and Donna was gracious about giving me a ride. On the way to the hotel, we found lots to talk about; and I felt so comfortable, I asked her to be my driver going back and forth for the rest of the retreat. I had another new friend. And I was proud of myself for being able to ask so many people for help.

———————————

12

Discover Vision Rehabilitation

HAVE YOU HEARD—OR THOUGHT "There is nothing more that can be done for your vision"? Those words can be devastating, especially when heard from an eye doctor, leaving one feeling scared, depressed, and hopeless. But in fact, there *is* something that can be done: VISION REHABILITATION.

What is vision rehabilitation?

Vision rehabilitation goes beyond the practical hints and strategies described in this book. It offers people with low vision specialized training in how to adjust to vision loss and use their remaining vision to maximize their daily functioning. Rehabilitation is provided by a variety of professionals in several kinds of organizations. Vision rehabilitation can help you develop a hopeful spirit, a sense of well-being, a personally satisfying level of independence, and an optimum quality of life—all leading to greater resiliency as you face new challenges.

Definition of low vision

According to the National Eye Institute, National Institutes of Health (National Eye Health Education Program), low vision is an impairment that is not correctable by standard eyeglasses, contact lenses, medication, or surgery, and that interferes with the ability to perform everyday activities, such as reading, shopping, cooking, writing, watching TV, recognizing faces, and seeing the color of clothes.

Who can benefit?

Anyone who experiences difficulty carrying out everyday tasks due to low vision qualifies for vision rehabilitation. People of all ages can be affected. Low vision can occur from birth defects, inherited diseases, injuries, diabetes, glaucoma, cataracts, and retinal diseases, including macular degeneration. Many older adults experience the effects of low vision from age-related diseases.

Professionals who offer rehabilitation

The primary medical specialist is the optometrist or ophthalmologist specializing in low vision. Many other types of specialists offer vision rehabilitation. Usually, a variety of professionals work in each rehabilitation organization. Staff may include vision rehabilitation therapists, occupational therapists, orientation and mobility trainers, counselors, cooking and skills trainers, and social workers.

Professional certification is available for some vision rehabilitation specialties. The Academy for Certification of Vision Rehabilitation and Education Professionals (ACVREP) offers both the Certified Vision Rehabilitation Therapist and the Certified Orientation and Mobility Specialist certificates. The American Occupational Therapy Association offers specialty certification in low vision.

Organizations offering vision rehabilitation

- Independent private agencies
- Private ophthalmology practices

- Private optometry practices

- State government agencies

- University Departments of Ophthalmology

- University Departments of Optometry

- Department of Veterans Affairs (ONLY for veterans of the US armed forces)

What services are offered?

Examples from the huge variety of services that may be offered by vision rehabilitation agencies are listed below, but not all organizations offer all of these services. (In some cases, a professional on staff is qualified to perform a complete vision examination.)

- Assistive devices training: Closed Circuit Television (CCTVs), magnifiers

- Cell smart phones: accessibility options, apps—finding and downloading, email sending and receiving, Internet access, making and receiving calls

- Community outreach presentations about services: assisted living and long-term care facilities; professional groups, such as occupational therapists; senior centers

- Computer accessibility training: email sending and receiving, keyboard typing skills, screen magnification software, screen reading software, voice recognition software

- Cooking: adaptive cooking and kitchen safety techniques, recipes in large type, special kitchen aids

- Counseling: counseling by staff members; one-on-one peer counseling with trained, visually impaired volunteers

- Electronic devices: ebook readers; tablet computers for reading, email, Internet

- Filling out forms: applications for Talking Books, applications for mobility services, income tax returns

- Finance management: banking, identifying money, paying bills, writing checks

- Fitness and health: designing a personalized fitness program, instruction on using fitness equipment, walking groups, yoga and workout classes

- Household management: marking and identifying clothing in closets, organizing household items and furniture

- In-home evaluation: developing a plan of service, identification of needs, information on community resources

- Job/vocational training and employment services

- Leisure and recreation: bingo, cribbage, and board games; book clubs; card games, such as hearts, bridge, and poker; craft classes, such as basket weaving, woodworking; journal and creative writing classes; lunch and supper club outings; movie showings with audio descriptions; needlework classes, such as knitting, crocheting; trips to museums and plays

- Library holdings: audio books, audio-described videos and DVDs, large print books and magazines

- Occupational therapy: driving interventions, home environment adaptations, mobility training, recreation and leisure activities, training in use of low vision devices

- Orientation and mobility training: instruction on the use of remaining vision and other senses, use of a white cane or a dog guide, depending on current vision, the ability to detect dangerous obstacles (such as stairs, curbs, moving vehicles, or people) in enough time to react safely

- Personal services, such as shopping assistance, pick-up and delivery, laundry

- Reading and listening: Braille instruction, Talking Books, radio and newspaper reading service, large print books and magazines

- Social workers: work with patients and their families to help adjustment to vision loss

- Support groups: led by a staff person or trained volunteer, meet others dealing with vision loss

- Transportation service: information on types of transportations services available in your community, especially those mandated by the Americans with Disabilities Act of 1990 (ADA), and assistance in filling out forms to obtain these services

- Volunteers and volunteering: help with shopping, reading, and leisure skills, opportunities to be a volunteer yourself!

- Youth services

When can I benefit?

There are no definite guidelines for when one should seek vision rehabilitation, and your doctor may not suggest it, so each person should be prepared to be a self-advocate. This can be a key to independence if you have reached the stage of "low vision," where it cannot be corrected by standard eyeglasses, medication, or surgery—and you are having problems performing your regular activities. Rehab can provide the skills to help a person with low vision remain safe, independent, and active at any stage of life.

How do I obtain services?

Optometrists and ophthalmologists specializing in low vision evaluate the need for vision rehabilitation and may recommend assistive devices. Sometimes referrals are made by ophthalmologists, retinologists, and/or occupational therapists. However, some clinicians may not be aware of the benefits of rehabilitation, so you may need to ask for a referral or be a self-advocate and contact the nearest rehabilitation organization.

What to expect from an evaluation

Specialized low vision testing techniques enable the doctor to obtain information about the nature and prognosis of the individual's eye disorder, corrected distance and near visual acuity, visual field status, focusing ability, range of eye movements, eye alignment, and depth perception discrimination. The doctor also evaluates the individual's color vision and ability to see low contrast objects.

At the completion of the evaluation, the doctor prescribes corrective lenses and adaptive devices that enable the individual to use their vision more effectively and efficiently for the specific activities they were having difficulty with, as well as for activities of daily living. The low vision clinician provides recommendations for appropriate size and contrast of reading materials, lighting and glare reduction strategies, magnification needs (including adaptive devices and technology), viewing strategies that will reduce the effects of central blind spots, as well as contrast enhancement strategies for both reading and writing activities. For individuals experiencing discomfort from outdoor glare, recommendations are made for specialty tints and glare-reducing coatings to increase contrast and comfort under glare or bright sunlit conditions.

Many communities have a vision loss agency that offers a wealth of services. Check the National Eye

Institute's list of resources. See Appendix B for description. [www.nei.nih.gov/lowvision/content/resources2.asp]

What is the cost?

Many nonprofit organizations offer free or low cost counseling and classes, plus a variety of recreational activities. Medicare may cover part of the cost of occupational therapy, but it must be ordered by a doctor and given by a Medicare provider.

Deciding to seek help

Some may find it intimidating to even think about looking for help outside a familiar environment. And, some people feel that they are surrendering independence by acknowledging the need for more help than friends and family can provide. Just the opposite is true. Learning new ways to navigate and understand low vision helps to maximize personal independence. Those who feel uncomfortable about the prospect of sharing their personal story with strangers, or about taking a class for the first time in years, will find that making that first call is a positive step. It shows that they are ready to open the door to whole new ways of living.

What will happen when I call?

The first step is to set up an appointment for an intake interview. If you have a referral document, bring it with you to the appointment. At this interview, basic identification information is gathered, and a discussion may cover the history of your vision loss. In some cases, a staff person also does a simple vision evaluation to get an idea of the equipment and services that might be helpful.

─────────── **MY STORY** ───────────

Finally!

I keep notes of every visit with my retinologist. Every now and then I made a note about a counselor at Vision Loss Resources, a local vision rehabilitation agency that my doctor mentioned on more than one visit. I had asked if there were any support groups, and the referral was in response to my question. I kept the idea of calling the counselor pretty well buried in the back of my mind until each time my retinologist brought it up again during subsequent visits. Still, I did nothing.

When I finally made the call to the counselor, I checked my notes and found that it had been four years since the doctor first told me about her. By then it had been eight years since my initial diagnosis.

The benefits of meeting with the counselor have been enormous. Perhaps the most important benefit is that, by taking that first step, I finally had become ready to go after help on my own.

At that first meeting, I kept hearing peals of laughter from the next room. I was then invited to join the group of men and women who were having a wonderful time eating the lunch that the cooking instructor had prepared in a demonstration. The people in this group had severe vision loss. I was seated next to two women who were members of the organization's advocacy group. Both were involved in community education. They went out to various facilities and told groups about the services offered by the center. The women also had received training to become paraprofessional aides to assist staff members who moderate support groups. These inspiring women showed me how much someone with severe macular disease could contribute, even when living with only peripheral vision.

Enrolling as a client at the center changed my life. My resolve to keep a positive outlook was affirmed and bolstered by meetings with my counselor. Other staff members have guided me in various ways. I have met inspiring people with vision loss in classes and at various functions at the center. In a weekly life skills class, I learned many new ways to live with vision loss, including special cooking techniques, how-to ideas for the all-important organization skills I need, and an upbeat approach to dealing with the frustrations of living with vision loss.

Why did I wait so long to take the first step in seeking help? My counselor told me that it was because I was not ready earlier. She said that people come at all stages of their vision loss. There is not a single "right" time for everyone. The right time is when one is ready. Sometimes I wish I had been ready earlier, but I think a streak of stubbornness got in my way. When others in my class who were at later stages of vision loss had difficulty reading the recipes printed in giant-size type, I kept thinking, "If only they had come sooner, they could have been using these practical ideas for years." Then I remembered that the same wisdom applied to me.

───────── **MY STORY** ─────────

Six Years Later

My vision continued to decline over the next six years. I decided it was time for me to have an examination by an optometrist expert in low vision rehabilitation who had been recommended to me. Another motivation was that I'd decided to write this new edition, and I wanted a firsthand experience of undergoing an examination by such a specialized optometrist.

This optometrist practices at the University of Iowa, so I made an appointment to see him when I was in Iowa City, visiting my daughter. I was comforted to have her wait with me before my appointment and to later find her waiting for me to hear the results.

The first step was by the technician who checked the prescriptions in both my reading and distance glasses. She asked if my eyes had been dilated recently, and when I told her yes, at my retinology appointment three weeks earlier, she was able to skip that step.

Then I was called into the doctor's examination room, I was surprised to see a new kind of eye chart. Instead of a chart with a large "E" on the top row and more and smaller letters on each succeeding row, the optometrist's chart had five large letters on the first row, and five smaller and smaller letters on each succeeding row. I've since learned that the chart I'd been accustomed to is called the Snellen chart, after its first developer in 1862. The chart with five letters across each line is called the ETDRS chart. It was developed in 1982 for the National Eye Institute for use in its Early Treatment Diabetic Retinopathy Study. I actually felt more relaxed reading the chart with the five letters per row than the one I was accustomed to for so many years with the large letter E on the top line.

Next was a test of my near vision. Remaining seated, I was handed a small card with several lines of a simple story where the lines of text became smaller and smaller. The strong light on the card came from a lamp behind me. As the lines became smaller, I twisted around in the chair to get closer to the light. Each line of the card indicated its size, such as 20/40. The doctor tested various lenses to see if a new prescription could help, but after doing a trial frame refraction, he said it was not possible to improve the prescriptions for either my distance or reading glasses.

Then we moved to another room that had a computer and a closed circuit television (called a CCTV and described in the next chapter, Embracing Technology). The CCTV looked like a computer with its monitor. The doctor started flashing different font samples in different sizes on the screen. Some were easier to read than others. It took several samples until we reached the one I could read easily. It was a plain non-serif font with no confusing curlicues. The biggest help was that the letters were white on a black background. I took the doctor's advice and have written this entire book with the letters in white on a black. The doctor advised updating my five-year-old computer to a new model with a 27" screen, advice I also followed. The doctor's parting words were that, considering I had lived with macular degeneration for thirteen years, I was doing very well.

———————————

13

Embrace Technology

FORGING AHEAD into the world of technology with an open mind can keep a person with low vision connected to the world and avoid the pitfalls of isolation. An array of assistive products are described in this chapter that offer new ways to help a person maintain current contacts and interests and develop new ones.

Technological products are valuable assistants in helping anyone operate at a maximum level of independence. There are people and organizations ready to help anyone who may be under the impression that these products are difficult to use. It's useful to explore and adopt the products that are the most helpful in any given situation.

Four categories of products are described in this chapter.

- Video magnification devices—handheld, portable, and desktop—that display enlarged images with adjustable contrast options

- Computers to connect to the Internet, use email, listen to music or audio books, view TV shows and movies, edit photos, and write documents

- Accessibility software for interacting with a computer by speaking and hearing.

- Mobile technology—phones and tablet computers for use away from home

(Audio technology for listening to books that are read aloud is covered in Chapter 4, Read to Expand Horizons.)

Video magnifiers

When an ordinary low-cost magnifying glass (some with LED lights) described on pages 47–48 no longer provides adequate help, it's time to consider electronic magnification.

Video magnifiers, sometimes called electronic magnifiers or CCTVs (closed circuit TVs), can enlarge images up to 68x in desktop models. They come in small portable handheld models as well as large stationary desktop sizes. A camera is used to take a photo of the material to be viewed and show a magnified image of that material on a screen. Varying levels of magnification are available within each unit, depending on the particular model. Most models show images in color—these are great for looking at photos.

There is a sharp difference in the cost of a video magnifier vs. a simple magnifying glass, with low-end video magnifiers costing well over a hundred dollars and high-end desktop magnifiers costing thousands of dollars. Models are described and shown in low vision catalogs. As part of vision rehabilitation, sometimes a prescription is given for a particular video device, such as a CCTV. These sometimes cost thousands of dollars, but some organizations can help defray the cost. State agencies for the blind and visually handicapped often provide them to those who meet eligibility requirements. See "Government agencies" in Appendix A. Rehabilitation provided through the Department of Veterans Affairs may cover the cost of the devices listed in this chapter.

Portable video magnifiers

Handheld electronic video magnifiers are made up of a camera and a built-in screen in the 4"–7" size range. Magnification levels are in the 2x to 24x range. The magnifiers are placed over the material to be viewed, and the image is displayed on the screen. These portable magnifiers are useful for reading print material, such as price tags, food labels at the grocery store, and menus at restaurants.

Desktop video magnifiers

This type of electronic magnifier looks like a computer because it has a monitor that is similar to a computer screen. In product catalogs, desktop video magnifiers are generally called CCTVs, or sometimes reading systems. Material is placed on a viewing table that is moved to position it by sliding the "XY" table side to side and up and down under the stationary video camera above the table. A magnified image of the text or photo is displayed on the screen. Screens are available in various sizes, and you can adjust the size of the magnification to meet your visual needs. Desktop magnifiers are useful for:

- reading documents, books, and newspapers.

- viewing photos.

- writing checks.

- recording deposits and withdrawals in a check register.

Magnifiers that plug into TVs or computers

With this "plug-and-play" video magnifier, a TV or computer monitor displays images, so the cost is much less than that of a desktop model. The device is actually a small handheld camera. To operate it, plug the cord of the device into the USB port of your computer or television set. Place the material you want to display on a table or desk, and move the device over the material. The camera scans the material and displays it on the screen in the magnification chosen from the options available with the specific brand and model. Handheld video magnifiers are useful for:

- reading documents, books, and newspapers.

- viewing photos.

Scanners convert text to speech

Unlike magnifiers that display images on a screen, scanner readers convert written material into spoken words by using OCR (optical character recognition) technology after a printed document is scanned by a camera. To operate this device, the reader is held over printed material and a button is pushed to snap a picture of the material. Next, OCR software converts the scanned image into recognized characters and words. Finally, a synthesizer speaks the recognized text.

Computer technology

For anyone not already using a computer, now is the time to start. Computers open up new worlds for writing, reading, speaking, and hearing, from keeping in touch with children and grandchildren by email to accessing the Internet and finding information on any topic. Anyone who is nervous about their ability to successfully navigate in the world of computers and related technology may be heartened to realize that many people with age-related eye diseases have had their first successful experiences with computers only after their vision loss. There are endless adaptive strategies for using a computer, including programs that read aloud the text that is displayed on the monitor.

Refresh typing skills

Those who are rusty at typing, or who use the hunt-and-peck system to select keyboard letters, can benefit from classes available in community education programs, senior centers, and other locations. Most people find they are better served by learning touch typing that trains the fingers to

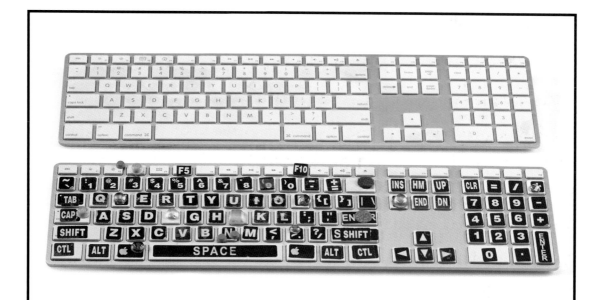

Regular keyboard and keyboard with large print, white-on-black stick-on labels

automatically go to the location of each key being sought. SeniorNet is a useful organization that offers both online and classroom courses in locations throughout the country. See Appendix B for more information.

For difficulty seeing the letters on the standard keyboard, large bold letters on stick-on labels can be applied to the keys. A more expensive option is a special keyboard with large, bold letters with black letters on white, black letters on yellow, or white letters on black. I started with a black-on-yellow keyboard; but when the keyboard on my new computer was not compatible, I found the stick-on labels worked even better. I use black on white, but other color combinations are also available.

Computers and monitors

For those who do not already own a computer, you may want to check with family members and friends before purchasing one. Someone may have an older model they are no longer using. The most important component is the monitor. Look for a model with a screen that can tilt backward because that position may make it easier to view text or images.

Computer accessibility options

Computers come with preinstalled accessibility options that help people with vision loss. Both PC Windows and Apple iMac computers offer useful standard options plus special accessibility tools.

Standard options

- Enlarge type size

- Select a readable font such as Calibri, Tahoma, or Verdana.

Special accessibility options

- Adjust contrast to change darkness of background

- Invert colors to white on black to provide greater contrast

- Magnifier to enlarge specific areas on the screen

- Adjust size and blink rate of cursor

- Speech recognition. The user does the talking into a microphone and the words appear on the screen as text. You can create documents, send email, and search the Internet. You do not need to use a keyboard.

- Screen reading/magnification. The computer talks through a speech synthesizer and reads aloud what is already on the screen. You select the reader from a selection of male and female voices.

Note that all Apple applications are available on iMac computers, iPhones, and iPads, and other Apple devices. See mobile technology section later in this chapter.

Advanced speech recognition and screen reading/ magnification software comes built into iMac computers, but advanced Windows software must be purchased separately as it does not come already installed on Windows computers. See Appendix B for list of brands and manufacturers.

Technology products

Most of the products described in this chapter are available from one or more of the low vision stores listed in Appendix A. Products are also available at electronics stores and from Internet sites. A list of representative manufacturers and US distributors is included in Appendix C. By visiting manufacturer websites, getting information over the phone, and visiting stores that sell these items, it is possible to learn about the latest products in the ever-changing field of assistive technology. Vision rehabilitation professionals are the best guides to finding what is right for you and helping you to obtain what you need.

The products mentioned in this chapter, unlike those discussed in other chapters, can cost hundreds and even thousands of dollars. If costs are prohibitive, it may be possible to get one or more of these products on loan, at a reduced cost, or even free through one of several organizations. Some of these organizations are listed below and described more fully in Appendix B. You need to meet financial and visual-impairment criteria, and you may be put on a waiting list because the products are often in short supply.

Each state has a commissioner for the blind who operates services for the blind and visually handicapped. See pages 232–234 for more information. Agencies usually have products on display. Home visits may be made by counselors to assess individual situations and determine whether or not a person qualifies for state services. Equipment that is given or loaned is brought to the person's home, and instructions are given on how to use each device.

Lions Clubs offer assistance in some communities. Veterans can receive rehabilitation services through the Department of Veterans Affairs, which has several programs that offer equipment and training. See Appendix A for contact information.

Electronic reading devices

An ebook (electronic version) or MP3 audio books are available for download from the Internet. See discussion at the end of Chapter 4.

Mobile technology

There are basic no-frills cell phones on the market that offer phone service and sometimes text messaging or cameras. They do not require data plans, and they cost less than multi-featured "smart" cell phones.

Smart phones and tablet computers offer access to email and the Internet while away from home. They perform most of the basic actions of a full-size desktop computer. There is a steady supply of new functions and applications.

Mobile cell phones

These smart phones come in two varieties, android phones, and iPhones made by Apple. Their functions are similar, but they have different operating systems and features. "Apps" is the name given to applications (called "software" or "programs" on computers).

Android and Apple smart phones

All the phones have touch screens. Android phones use the Google operating system. They are made by several different manufacturers and come in many different models, accessibility features, and applications. The iPhone accessibility options have different names from the android models.

Here is a list of helpful features and built-in accessibility options that variously come with smart phones. At the end is a list of apps that can be downloaded.

- **Screen reader.** Announces who is calling, reads email and text messages, describes what is happening on the screen, and announces what is on web pages. Earphones can be used in public for listening to emails and texts.

- **Dictation.** Converts spoken words and numbers into text and types emails and URLs.

- **Personal intelligent assistant.** Assists with any questions about anything—places phone calls, sends messages, identifies your exact location, checks for movies, suggests a nearby restaurant, and can be used to listen to music, check flights, and interact with social networks.

- **Large text.** Increases font size up to 56 points. When activated, all text on the phone is enlarged.

- **Invert colors.** Changes text to black type on a white background. The greater contrast makes words easier to see and read.

Mark's favorite apps

My friend Mark, from our local chapter of the Foundation Fighting Blindness, shared his favorite iPhone apps that make it possible for him to work and navigate even with very limited central vision from Stargardt disease.

Built-in apps

- Clock, timer, and alarm: The clock automatically announces the time with the touch of a button.

The timer and alarm clock are easily set by voice command. When cooking—no need to deal with the timer on the oven.

- When unable to respond to a message by voice, he uses a small Bluetooth (wireless) keyboard; when typing, the phone reads back what is being typed.

- Typing is easier when he inverts colors to white on black and enlarges the type size.

- Stock market and weather updates are built-in apps that can be customized to give updates on whatever you to want to know.

- Internet websites can be verbally accessed. Once a website pops up, it takes just a few finger clicks to hear information.

Downloadable apps

- NEWSLINE®, a free service of the National Federation for the Blind, makes over 300 newspapers available. The Voiceover screen reader makes it easy to navigate through the sections and to find an article.

- Flashlight turns the camera flash into a bright flashlight.

- Money Reader shows the phone any type of currency and announces the denomination.

- Skype makes it possible to see the person you are talking with.

- DropBox allows viewing of files from home location, eliminating the need to bring a laptop when traveling.

- Airline travel is easier at major airports that accept your boarding pass that has been sent to your phone. No more paper boarding passes!

Mark is able to perform all these functions using speech commands, as he is not able to read the screen.

Tablet computers

Tablet computers are essentially designed to bridge the gap in mobile computing between traditional laptops and smart phones. They are lightweight and portable, but the screens are large enough to be easy to see and read. Screen sizes range from 13" down to minis at 5". Most models will fit in a purse or briefcase. Weights range from 8 to 2 pounds. Prices are in between those of smart phones and desktop computers.

Tablet computers offer the same features as smart phones—minus the phone. Their larger screens make it easier to read articles, download and read ebooks and MP3 audio books, view TV shows and movies, and play games. Banks offer apps that allow banking services, including access to balances, bill paying, funds transfers, and check deposits made by taking a picture of the check with the tablet's camera.

New developments

The newest developments in 2013 included wearable technology—smart watches and glasses that perform mobile computing. Several companies offered smart watches with features such as GPS, heart monitors, cameras, and Wi-Fi. Smart glasses combined a camera, display, touchpad, battery, and microphone. These features are built into spectacle frames, so displays are placed in front of the eyes. The glasses can alert users to emails, text messages, and phone calls. Music from websites can be remotely controlled.

Certainly, new assistive technologies will continue to be developed to bring greater independence to those with vision loss.

14

Research Changes the Future

RESEARCH HAS BROUGHT US to treatments and cures for a host of eye diseases. Throughout the world, individual and university research centers and institutes are funded by government agencies, public-private partnerships, private fundraising organizations, and personal philanthropy. Following are a few examples.

National Eye Institute, National Institutes of Health

"Research Today, Vision Tomorrow" is the banner headline on the website homepage of the National Eye Institute, a division of the National Institutes of Health. NEI was established in 1968 by Public Law

90-489. It was the first government organization solely dedicated to research on human visual diseases and disorders. NEI officially began operations on December 26, 1968, and its mission is to "conduct and support research, training, health information dissemination, and other programs with respect to blinding eye diseases, visual disorders, mechanisms of visual function, preservation of sight, and the special health problems and requirements of the blind."

In 2011 the NEI awarded more than 1,400 grants to organizations such as universities and small businesses. In 2013 the NEI identified the goal to "Regenerate Neurons and Neural Connections in the Eye and Visual System," including—

- Molecular Therapy for Eye Disease
- Intersection of Aging & Biological Mechanisms of Eye Disease

Broad areas of NEI funded research—

- Retinal diseases
- Corneal diseases
- Lens and cataracts

- Glaucoma and optic neuropathies

- Strabismus, amblyopia, and visual processing

- Low vision and blindness

THE NEI sponsors clinical trials—medical research studies in which people volunteer to participate—to evaluate the safety and effectiveness of a new procedure, medication, or device to prevent, diagnose, or treat an eye disease or disorder. Generally, medical research begins in laboratories. After a treatment shows promise in the laboratory, it is tested in a study to determine if it will be beneficial for patients. You can let your doctor know that you would be interested in participating if a trial is starting for your disease. The first thing I did after my diagnosis was to join a five-year study on laser treatment for macular degeneration, and knowing that I was in a research study helped me develop my positive attitude.

Foundation Fighting Blindness (FFB)

Founded in 1971, the FFB states in its 2012 annual report. "The urgent mission of the Foundation Fighting Blindness, Inc. is to drive the research that will provide preventions, treatments, and cures for people affected by retinal disease."

FFB funds research in areas such as genetics, gene therapy, retinal cell transplantation, regenerative medicine, novel medical therapies, cellular and molecular mechanisms, pharmaceutical and nutritional therapies, and clinical, or human, trials which help determine the safety and efficacy of potential treatments.

Disease categories of 2012 FFB grants:

- Macular degeneration: AMD, Best disease, Stargardt disease

- Leber congenital amaurosis

- Retinitis pigmentosis

- Usher syndrome

- Rare diseases including : Bardet-biedl syndrome, choroideremia, retinoschisis, and the entire spectrum of retinal degenerative diseases

FFB's research effort is global. In 2012 the foundation was funding 123 projects at 76 research institutions around the world, including those in the United

States, England, France, Germany, the Netherlands, Israel, and China.

Since its inception, FFB has raised more than $450 million. Through its fifty volunteer chapters across the United States, FFB raises funds through its annual VisionWalks and Dining in the Dark dinners, held annually in member cities. Through these events, the volunteers both raise money for research and increase public awareness of vision loss.

Private philanthropy—Wynn gift

A major gift was made to the University of Iowa's Institute for Vision Research in August 2013. The twenty-five-million-dollar commitment by Stephen Wynn will be used to accelerate progress toward cures for rare, inherited retinal diseases. Mr. Wynn knows firsthand what it is like to lose vision from a rare inherited eye disease, retinitis pigmentosa. He stated, "I am thrilled by the pace of the scientific progress that has occurred in the past few years, and I feel that the prospect of finding a cure is possible and probable in the short term and certain in the long term." He said he selected the University of

Iowa because of its "army of clinicians and scientists who have uncovered many of the secrets of the genome and are now on the cusp of applying them in the clinic." The gift will help maintain the valuable collaborative relationships that have been developed with other vision scientists around the world.

Mr. Wynn said, "My support is given on behalf of the millions of people worldwide who awaken every day to a dark world . . . None of us will rest until the lights are back on for everyone."

My outlook

I am inspired and encouraged by the efforts made by so many to "keep the lights on" for all of us. In the introduction to this book, I said my goal is to offer the hope that leads to an independent and fulfilling life.

I keep hope by remembering that there will always be one more thing to try.

I live with hope, and you can, too!

Appendix A

Low Vision Stores

ALMOST ALL of the products mentioned in this book are available at the low vision stores listed below and online. There may be local stores in your community where you can also see and obtain some of the products.

LS&S

1808-G Janke Drive, Northbrook, IL 60062

800-468-4789

www.lssproducts.com

Maxi-Aids, Inc.

42 Executive Boulevard, Farmingdale, NY 11735

800-522-6294

www.maxiaids.com

Appendix B

National Information Resources

NATIONAL ORGANIZATIONS DEVOTED TO helping individuals and their families adapt to living with vision loss provide up-to-date information through their websites and newsletters. They offer services in the areas of advocacy, education, research, fundraising, and local chapters. Although some have the word "Blind" in their names, they are for anyone with vision loss. Some agencies have changed their name to reflect that broader community. The following list of selected organizations is divided into private nonprofit organizations and government agencies.

Private Nonprofit Organizations

American Foundation for the Blind (AFB)

800-232-5463

www.afb.org

Newsletter: VisionAware

Founded in 1921, AFB works to ensure that the rights and interests of people with vision loss are represented in public policies and that they have access to the information, technology, education, and legal resources needed to live independent and productive lives.

The AFB main website features comprehensive profiles of agencies and descriptions of all the services they offer. FamilyConnect is a website for families of children with visual impairments that is sponsored by AFB and the National Association for Parents of Children with Visual Impairments (NAPVI), listing agencies that offer services for children and describing those services. VisionAware with SeniorSite is AFB's website for adults and seniors with visual impairments, listings agencies that offer services for adults and seniors and describing those services.

The AFB directory contains information on more than 2,000 organizations and agencies in the government and private, nonprofit sectors that provide a wide variety of direct and indirect services, information, and other assistance. Information is also included on producers and distributors of Braille, large print publications, audiotapes, and other alternate media; specialized computer hardware and software and other assistive technology, and reviews of assistive and household products.

American Macular Degeneration Foundation (AMDF)

888-622-8527
www.macular.org
Find an eye care professional
www.macular.org/proffeye.html
Find a state agency:
www.macular.org/stagency.html
Canadian services: International services:
www.macular.org/internat.html
Publication: www.macular.org/spotlite.html

The AMDF newsletter *SPOTLIGHT* provides scientific information, including recent research. The American

Macular Degeneration Foundation works for the prevention, treatment, and cure of macular degeneration by raising funds, educating the public, and supporting scientific research. Directories by state include topics such as state agencies, low vision centers, and eye care professionals.

American Occupational Therapy Association, Inc. (AOTA)

301-652-2682

www.aota.org

AOTA is an official association of occupational therapists in the United States. The goals of its low vision specialty are to prevent accident and injury, teach new skills, and promote a healthy and satisfying lifestyle. Services of an occupational therapist generally require a referral from a doctor. These professionals offer rehabilitation training in the areas of cooking, marking items for easy identification, developing senses besides sight, and using assistive devices. These services are provided in your home, and suggestions may be made about your lighting and furniture arrangements.

Better Health for Better Vision

www.WebRN-MacularDegeneration.com

Newsletter: Macular Degeneration News

Newsletter archive: www.webrn-macular
degeneration.com/WebRNMacular
_Degeneration_News-backissues.html

The goal of the health and technology oriented weekly email newsletter, *Macular Degeneration News*, and its website is to raise awareness and knowledge of macular degeneration. By covering topics such as the risks, causes, symptoms, and treatment of macular degeneration, it works to bring hope to those who have been diagnosed with the disease. There is special emphasis on new assistive products and on medical advances, research and clinical trials, diet and supplements; and helpful aids, such as many types of magnifiers.

Foundation Fighting Blindness (FFB)

800-683-5555

www.blindness.org

The mission of the FFB is to drive research that leads to the prevention, treatment, and cure of retinal disease. More than fifty volunteer-led chapters raise funds, increase public awareness, hold educational meetings, and provide support to each other and their communities.

FFB has funded thousands of research studies in promising areas such as genetics, gene therapy, retinal cell transplantation, artificial retinal implants, and pharmaceutical and nutritional therapies. The FFB provides information and outreach programs for patients, families, and professionals. The website lists current clinical trials and features pages on retinitis pigmentosa, macular degeneration, Usher syndrome, and a large spectrum of other retinal degenerative diseases. *InFocus*, mailed three times a year to members, reports on research, science news, and FDA-approved clinical trials.

International Association of Audio Information Services (IAAIS)

800-280-5325
www.iaais.org/index.html

The IAAIS is a worldwide volunteer-driven organization of over a hundred independent Audio Information Services that turn text into speech for those who are unable to read or hold printed material. Most services use volunteer readers, and many US stations are associated with public radio stations, colleges and universities, and libraries. The IAAIS website offers a large type option and includes a directory of radio stations that provide immediate, verbatim audio access to newspapers, magazines, consumer information, and selected material such as public affairs programs, books, and daily exercise programs.

Some services also offer a variety of related programs, such as personal reader programs; audio-description services of live theater, museum exhibits, nature trails, parades, and other visual venues; audio transcription; taping services; and other audio-based community services.

Lions Clubs International

630-468-6901
www.lionsclubs.org

Lions Club International has over 46,000 clubs and 1.35 million members, making it the world's largest service club organization. The website, offered in a multitude of languages, includes a Find a Club link.

For nearly 100 years, its members have worked to prevent blindness, restore eyesight and improve eye care for hundreds of millions of people worldwide. Local clubs sponsor programs for the visually impaired and donate aids such as talking clocks and, sometimes, computers to people who are visually impaired. Some clubs provide large print books to libraries. Lions Club services include supporting guide dog schools, scholarships for blind students and vocational training programs, facilitating self-help groups, and supporting recreational activities and Lions camps for the blind/visually impaired.

Macular Degeneration Partnership

310-623-4466
www.amd.org

AMD News Update, an email newsletter, features information regarding current research on both the dry and wet forms of macular degeneration. The newsletter also is in easy to read white on black with yellow banners.

The Macular Degeneration Partnership is an outreach program of the nonprofit Discovery Eye Foundation with a mission to provide comprehensive, easily understood, and up-to-the-minute information about macular degeneration to the public through the Internet, telephone, public events, and printed materials. The organization's goal is to support research and coordinate advocacy efforts.

Macular Disease Society (UK)

0300 3030 111

www.maculardisease.org

This British organization is the national charity for anyone affected by central vision loss. With more than 15,000 members it's the biggest UK patient group in the sight loss sector, and the voice of people with macular conditions.

The society is dedicated to providing information and practical support so that those with macular disease may make the most of their remaining vision. The informative website reports on promising research, promotes independence, confidence, and quality of life; promotes and funds research into macular degeneration; and hosts a discussion forum for its members, covering many topics.

National Association for Parents of Children with Visual Impairments (NAPVI)

www.spedex.com/napvi

The NAPVI is a nonprofit organization of, by, and for parents committed to providing support to the parents of children who have visual impairments. NAPVI is a core partner for the Families & Advocates Partnership for Education (FAPE) project spearheaded by the Parent Advocacy Coalition for Education Rights (PACER).

NAPVI and AFB offer an online multimedia community, called Family Connect [http://www.familyconnect.org], for parents and guardians of children with vision impairments.

National Federation of the Blind (NFB)

www.nfb.org
410-659-9314

The NFB is an advocacy association with chapters around the country. Founded in 1940, the Federation has grown to over 50,000 members in over seven hundred local chapters. The NFB advocates for the civil rights and equality of blind Americans and develops innovative education, technology, and training programs to provide the blind, and those who are losing vision, with the tools they need to become independent and successful.

NFB offers the free NFB-NEWSLINE® to those who cannot read regular newsprint. Over 300 newspapers are available. Information is available at www.nfb.org/audio-newspaper-service or by calling 1-866-504-7300.

Prevent Blindness America (PBA)

800-331-2020
www.preventblindness.org

Founded in 1908, PBA is a volunteer eye health and safety organization whose mission is to prevent blindness and preserve sight. The organization offers education programs, screenings for vision problems in adults at locations such as senior centers and for children in schools, and various community and patient service programs. The website lists affiliates in the states where they are available. PBA advocates at the local, state, and national levels to promote sound public policy and adequate funding for initiatives that prevent blindness and save sight.

PBA also provides funding for scientists who will find tomorrow's cures for the eye diseases that threaten vision loss and blindness.

SeniorNet

571-203-7100

www.seniornet.org

Founded in 1986, SeniorNet's mission is to provide older adults with education and access to computer technologies to enhance their lives and enable them to share their knowledge and wisdom. As a national nonprofit organization with international affiliates, SeniorNet is funded by membership dues, Learning Center fees, the altruistic donations of individuals and the generous support and sponsorship of corporations and foundations.

The organization publishes a newsletter and supports about 200 Learning Centers throughout the US and in other countries. The website provides a list of these centers, organized by state and country. Training is available to those new to using a computer, and for those who wish to improve existing skills, to prepare for new employment, or to use the Internet.

Government Agencies

The Assistive Technology Act, commonly known as the "Tech Act," was enacted by Congress in 1998 to fund general types of programs, which vary from state to state, such as grant programs, protection and advocacy services, and alternative financing programs for purchasing assistive technology. The Tech Act provides lifelong services to those who live with any type of disability.

Some government agencies have special programs for people who are eligible for services if they meet the agencies' strict definition of "blind."

Department of Veterans Affairs, VHA Optometry Service, Low Vision Rehabilitation

www.va.gov/BLINDREHAB/VIST.asp
202-461-7317

Veterans and eligible active duty service members should contact the VIST coordinator in the VA facility nearest their home or the Blind Rehabilitation Service Program office at 202-461-7317. The VHA Optometry Service offers a wide variety of services along the continuum of visual impairment, ranging from primary eye and low vision care to programs at the Visual Impairment Center and Optimize Remaining Sight (VICTORS) and Blind Rehabilitation Centers (BRCs). Optometrists help visually impaired veterans maintain functionality and independence by diagnosing levels of decreased vision and prescribing low vision devices, such as specialized lens designs and prescriptions, pocket and handheld magnifiers, prismatic eyeglasses, telescopes, special lighting, and non-optical devices such as closed circuit televisions (CCTVs) and head-mounted displays.

Internal Revenue Service

800-829-1040

www.irs.gov/publications/p554/ch04.html

If you meet IRS criteria for eligibility, you can receive an income tax deduction for blindness that is equal to the deduction for being over sixty-five years old. To claim the deduction for "partly blind," you must have a statement certified by your eye doctor or registered optometrist that declares one of the following:

- Even with glasses or contact lenses, you cannot see better than 20/200 in your better eye, or;
- Your field of vision is 20 degrees or less.

Medicare and Medicaid Services (Centers for)

800-633-4227

Organizational phone list at www.cms.hhs.gov

Services covered by Medicare depend on the specific plan you have and whether or not you are also covered by Medicaid. Coverage varies from plan to plan, but services may include doctor visits, prescription drug coverage, coverage of costs incurred with eye injections, surgery for drooping eyelids or eyebrows, and mobility training. Check with your provider for information on the vision-related services that are covered in your plan.

National Eye Institute (NEI)

301-496-5248

www.nei.nih.gov

The NEI was founded by Congress in 1968. It is part of the National Institutes of Health. The NEI is the major source in the US for information about eye diseases and funding research to find treatments and cures. See Chapter 15 for NEI research activities.

The NEI website provides comprehensive information, including a list of eye diseases and disorders, a list of clinical studies, and free publications.

The National Eye Health Education Program (NEHEP) was established to increase awareness of scientifically based health information that can be applied to preserving sight and preventing blindness. NEHEP works in partnership with public and private organizations that conduct eye health education programs. NEHEP promotes early detection and timely treatment of eye disease and the use of vision rehabilitation services, providing healthcare professionals with information, materials, and resources to educate patients and the public about eye health and the importance of comprehensive dilated eye examinations.

National Council of State Agencies for the Blind (NCASB)

717-783-3784
www.ncsab.org

The mission of the NCSAB is to promote, through advocacy, coordination, and education, the delivery of specialized services that enable individuals who are blind and visually impaired to achieve personal and vocational independence. NCSAB serves agencies in each state that meet the needs of the blind and visually handicapped, providing a directory and a forum for its members. The agencies have various names, including State Services for the Blind and Visually Handicapped; Blind Services, Department of Human Services; Aid to the Aged, Blind or Disabled; and Board of Education and Services for the Blind.

Each state provides services to the visually handicapped, but the government organizations themselves and the services they provide vary from state to state.

Services can include:

- Vocational rehabilitation and job placement services
- Financial assistance or referrals to other agencies and organizations that provide similar services in the community

- Orientation and mobility training and transportation

- Communication center with a special library and transcription service, providing reading material in alternate formats to citizens who have difficulty reading normal print

- Provision of playback machines for the Talking Book program

Appendix C

Manufacturers of Technology Products

THE TECHNOLOGY PRODUCTS described in Chapter 13 are generally available from the low vision stores. Assistive technology is developing at such a rapid pace that information on specific products is soon outdated. Thus the list here includes manufacturers and their websites, with a note of their general types of products.

Ai Squared

www.aisquared.com

Software for screen reading (ZoomText) and screen magnification

Dolphin Computer Access, Ltd.

www.yourdolphin.com

Software for screen reading and screen
magnification

Enhanced Vision

www.enhancedvision.com

Portable and desktop video magnifiers

Freedom Scientific

www.freedomscientific.com

Handheld video magnifiers and screen reading and
magnification software (MAGic)

Guerilla Technologies

www.guerillatechnologies.com

Software for text to speech, with screen
magnification

Human Ware

www.humanware.com

Handheld and desktop magnifiers

Nuance

www.nuance.com

Software for speech recognition (Dragon)

Optelec

www.optelec.com

Desktop and portable video magnifiers (CCTVs)

Serotek Corporation

www.serotek.com

Software for text to speech, with screen
magnification

About this book's design

THIS TRULY LARGE PRINT BOOK was designed specifically for the reader with limited vision. The book is printed on glare-resistant, heavy paper that makes the pages durable and easy to turn. The off-white color provides good contrast against the large, heavy, black type.

My goal was to use a font that is easy to read, along with a layout that has clearly identified topics. This book is in a sans serif font. Serifs are small decorative embellishments to individual letters and numerals that can distract the eye when trying to distinguish letters. The more open sans serif fonts are easier for people with low vision to read. Consider the difficulty you may have in knowing whether a numeral is a 6 or a 9 because the loops are almost closed. In the open font of this book, it is easier to distinguish the two numbers than it is in many serif fonts.

To choose an easy-to-read sans serif font, several were tested with low vision readers who were members of support groups. This Frutiger font was named the winner. Designed by Adrian Frutiger for signage in the Charles de Gaulle airport in Paris, where the installation was completed in 1975, the font is known for its legibility.

To find a layout that would clearly identify topics, several versions were tested. The low vision readers preferred large headings that indicate new topics. They were quite firm about placing the page numbers at the bottom of the page, in the center.

The designer and the author hope that you enjoy handling and reading this book.

Acknowledgments

I am grateful for the support, encouragement, and information I received as I undertook this complete revision of my earlier books titled *Macular Disease, Practical Strategies for Living with Vision Loss*.

My thanks to the inspiring members of the Minnesota chapter of the Foundation Fighting Blindness for expanding my understanding of the vast world of vision loss, with acknowledgment to Mark Valenziano for his contribution on apps.

Thanks also to the staff at Vision Loss Resources in Minneapolis, and to participants in my classes and presentations, and to Mark E. Wilkinson, OD, from the University of Iowa.

I thank my talented publishing team whose professionalism led to the previous edition of this book winning first place in two prestigious book competitions. Thank you to editor and collaborator Marly Cornell, designer Monica Baziuk, photographer

Scott Knutson, indexer Galen Schroeder, and proofreader Rosemary Kokesh.

My heartfelt gratitude to my family for their support from the moment I had the idea of writing the first edition of this book—my daughter Katie Wolfe; my sister Jean Richter; and my son Steven Wolfe, for buying and installing products I tested for this book, his assistance and ideas at the photo shoot, and for contributing "My Son's Story." To my late husband, Fancher E. Wolfe, my most poignant thanks for so much.

About the author

PEGGY R. WOLFE is uniquely qualified to write a book about living with vision loss. Her expertise with macular disease dates back to the 1950s when her uncle became legally blind and she read aloud his favorite books. In the early 1980s, her mother discovered after cataract surgery that the underlying cause of her vision loss was macular degeneration. Peggy helped by writing checks, shopping, errands, companionship, and placing orders for her mother's beloved Talking Books. Then, in 1999, at the age of sixty-nine, Peggy was diagnosed with macular degeneration.

Writing a book about what she has learned, and continues to learn, was a natural choice. Peggy's father authored how-to books on electrical wiring, and she serves as the president of the publishing company he founded in 1939. An English and philosophy major in college, she earned a master's degree in library science. She established the corporate library at the Pillsbury Company and later worked as a research fellow/librarian at the University of Minnesota.

Peggy lives in Minnetonka, Minnesota, volunteers in her church's music department, takes ballet classes through her school district's adult enrichment program, and studies Pilates and kettlebells with private instructors. She has given presentations on vision loss at senior centers and taught short courses in community education programs. When Peggy celebrated her eightieth birthday in 2010 at a surprise birthday party in ballet class, she was inspired to dance across the floor, shouting her new slogan, "Eighty Power!"

Index

■ M

■ S

Vision rehabilitation, continued

　　　　organizations offering, 177–178, 182

　　　　services provided, 178–181

Vitamins, 25–27

Vocational training, 180, 224, 232–233

Voice recognition, 179, 199–200

Voice synthesizer, 196, 200

Volunteering, 11–13, 181, 213, 222

■ **W**

White cane, 150, 180

Order Book

Call 1-800-841-0383, or send check, money order, or credit card information (VISA, MasterCard, American Express, or Discover) to:

Park Publishing, Inc.
511 Wisconsin Drive
New Richmond, WI 54017-2613
Fax 715-246-4366
Email parkpublishing@nrmsinc.com

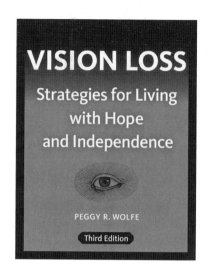

PRICE PER COPY	COPIES
$19.95 + $3.50 shipping	Single
$15.95 + shipping (by wgt)	2–5
$13.95 + shipping (by wgt)	6–10
$11.95 + shipping (by wgt)	11–50

For over 50 copies, call 1-800-841-0383 for discounts.

Please send the following, based on above discounts.

#_____ copies @ $_____ = $_____

Minnesota residents add 6.875% sales tax.
Shipping by UPS Ground will be added for two or more copies.
(Call 1-800-841-0383 for shipping quote.)

Name _____

Address _____

City _____ State _____ ZIP _____

Phone _____ Email _____

Credit card information
Name on card _____

Card number _____ Exp _____ / _____

Security code _____